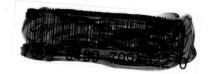

D1573340

the real
body
manual

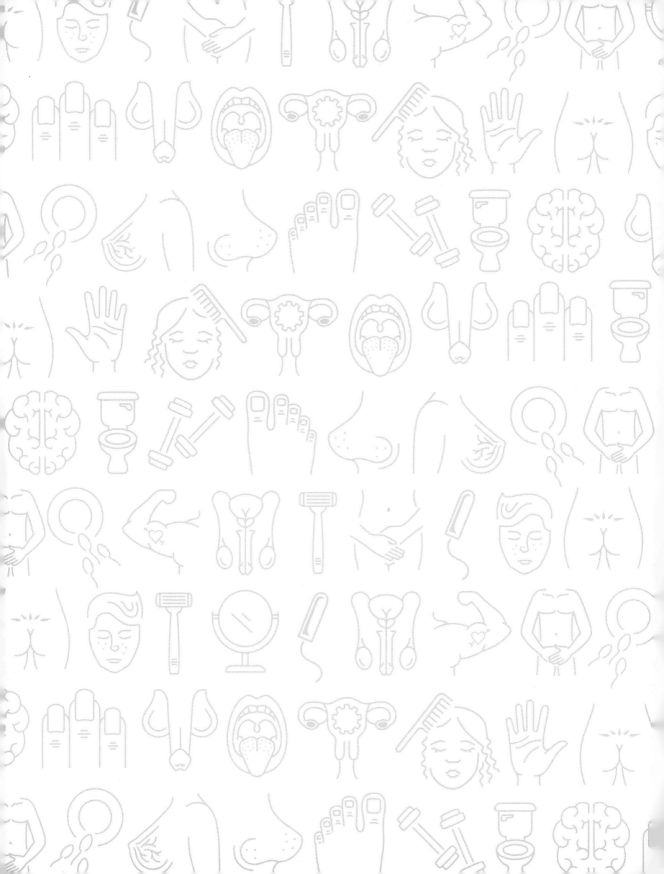

the real body manual

YOUR VISUAL GUIDE

TO HEALTH & WELLNESS

NANCY REDD

Avery

an imprint of Penguin Random House

New York

AVERY

an imprint of Penguin Random House LLC
penguinrandomhouse.com

Most Avery books are available at special quantity discounts for bulk purchase for sales promotions, premiums, fundraising, and educational needs. Special books or book excerpts also can be created to fit specific needs. For details, write SpecialMarkets@penguinrandomhouse.com.

Library of Congress Cataloging-in-Publication Data

Names: Redd, Nancy, author.
Title: The real body manual: your visual guide to health & wellness / Nancy Redd.
Description: New York: Avery, an imprint of Penguin Random House, [2024] | Includes index. |
    Audience: Ages 12+
Identifiers: LCCN 2023053371 (print) | LCCN 2023053372 (ebook) | ISBN 9780593541401
    (trade paperback) | ISBN 9780593541418 (ebook)
Subjects: LCSH: Body image in adolescence—Juvenile literature. | Teenagers—Health and hygiene—
    Juvenile literature. | Adolescent psychology—Juvenile literature.
Classification: LCC BF724.3.B55 R43 2024 (print) | LCC BF724.3.B55 (ebook) | DDC 306.4/613—dc23/
    eng/20231214
LC record available at https://lccn.loc.gov/2023053371
LC ebook record available at https://lccn.loc.gov/2023053372

Printed in China
10 9 8 7 6 5 4 3 2 1

Book and cover design by Ashley Tucker

For August and Nancy Rupali,
the best kids a mom could ask for. Thank you
for encouraging me to write this manual for y'all—
the process has made me a wiser person and a better parent!

contents

introduction:

let's get real!

Why aren't humans born with a body manual? Wouldn't it make sense for all of us to enter this world with a bunch of instructions attached to our umbilical cords? After all, every other important item in our lives comes with at least a little FYI, from our favorite jeans (check the tag) to our beloved smartphones (check the box). Even microwave pizza comes with a few directions, and I think we can all agree that our bodies are more complicated than frozen food!

Unlike clothes and electronics, you don't outgrow or upgrade yourself. We all get one body that carries us through this complicated life from beginning to end, and it's essential to figure out how to love, troubleshoot, and take care of it as best we can. This can feel like a struggle sometimes, can't it?

It's always been a challenge—take it from me. Growing up, I hated my body. I was embarrassed by and ashamed of how it looked and smelled, and sometimes by how it felt. I didn't know how to tell when something was wrong or not, when to go to the doctor to seek help, or even how to ask for advice in the first place! Over many years, I discovered that most of what I stressed about was totally common, and some issues I assumed were okay actually required medical attention.

At Harvard, I was lucky enough to major in women's studies, and I spent quite a few years as a young adult examining the many ways that our society tends to normalize body shaming, inventing "problems" that make many of us feel insecure enough to obsess over expensive and time-consuming ways to fix these so-called problems that society made up. It's quite the annoying cycle! And yet, here I was, fresh out of puberty and armed with loads of knowledge but *still* feeling bodily shame. All this frustration and confusion led me to start writing about the human body in realistic, matter-of-fact ways to help us all separate the realities of our physical bodies from unrealistic societal expectations.

Today, I have two wonderful kids entering puberty themselves—August (he/him) and my namesake, Li'l Nancy (she/her). To my delight, they're asking many of the same questions I had growing up, and I'm so excited to support them as much as I can. It's been well over a decade since I've written about or even thought seriously about coming-of-age, so to help navigate this stage of life, I went searching for modern resources for our family chats and my kids' nightstands. I've bought many wonderfully written books, some with mind-blowingly amazing illustrations, but I was surprised to see that after all this time, none of them had pictures of real body parts. After all, if there's one thing I've learned after writing about body image and self-esteem for over two decades, with a few photographic health books under my belt, it's that seeing is believing, and having authentic, unaltered photos to compare and contrast with one's own body can make all the difference when it comes to a person's comfort with and capacity to handle their common and not-so-common concerns.

So, as I tend to do whenever there's a resource that I or my kids need that I can't find, I decided to create one myself! With the help of a bunch of brilliant medical experts, I'm proud that *The Real Body Manual* is factual, friendly, and full of instructions—just like a manual should be. Plus, thanks to dozens of brave and bold humans (and the fantastic Brynne Zaniboni behind the lens), this manual is uniquely photographic, making it the perfect love letter to the type of adults I hope my children become—informed, open-minded, body confident, and, most importantly, *real*.

But this manual is not just a gift for my children—I also wrote it for all of *you*. That's why it's YOUR photographic guide to health and wellness, because the more we know about every human body, the better care we can take of ourselves and our fellow humans.

If your specific lived experience is missing from this manual, know that it's only omitted from these few pages and not from my heart—your perspective is valuable and valid. My dream would be for *The Real Body Manual* to have a thousand pages and two thousand photos, but that would have broken the printing press (and bookshelves). While this manual is packed with photos, and its words have been reviewed by a number of medical professionals, parents, and other people from many walks of life, it isn't comprehensive. Rather, it strives to be a nonjudgmental, shame-free, and thought-provoking conversation starter.

The Real Body Manual is designed for you to crack open anytime and turn to any page to learn something new about the body. It's here to help any curious person get on the right path to understanding how bodies work, become comfortable chatting with a medical professional if something seems off, and feel capable of advocating for yourself—and others—on the never-ending journey toward health and happiness.

I hope it helps!

Love, Nancy Redd (she/her)

PLEASE NOTE:

This manual uses inclusive language to affirm the millions of people who are intersex as well as all gender identities.

The descriptor "people" is used throughout instead of the gender binary terms of "guys" or "girls" because humans aren't that simple.

Likewise, this manual uses "people born with penises" and "people born with vaginas" and acknowledges genital diversity and uniqueness when discussing maturation-based physical changes to the body.

Occasionally, when talking about genitalia, this manual uses "people with penises" and "people with vaginas" because many people who are transgender or have intersex variations aren't born with the genitalia they die with.

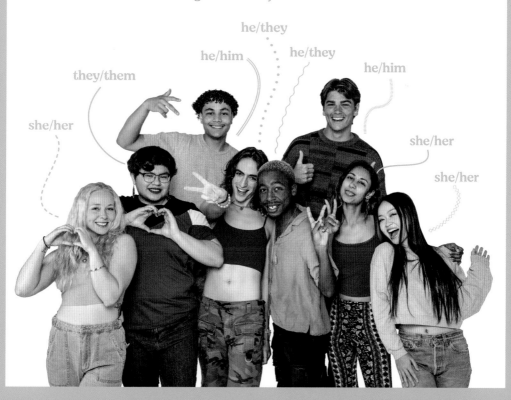

body skin

&

facial skin

You should really try to love the skin you're in . . . because there's a lot of it! Skin is the body's largest, heaviest, and fastest-growing organ. About 15 percent of your body weight is skin, so if you weigh 140 pounds, over 20 pounds is skin!

Skin is our body's armor, protecting us and our vital organs from injury.

Our skin has many functions, including:

+ Shielding our bodies from injury, infection, and UV rays

+ Regulating body temperature and preventing dehydration

+ Enabling us to feel pain, warmth, cold, pressure, and other sensations

+ Producing hormones crucial to our health, like vitamin D

+ Storing water, fat, and other products our bodies need to function properly

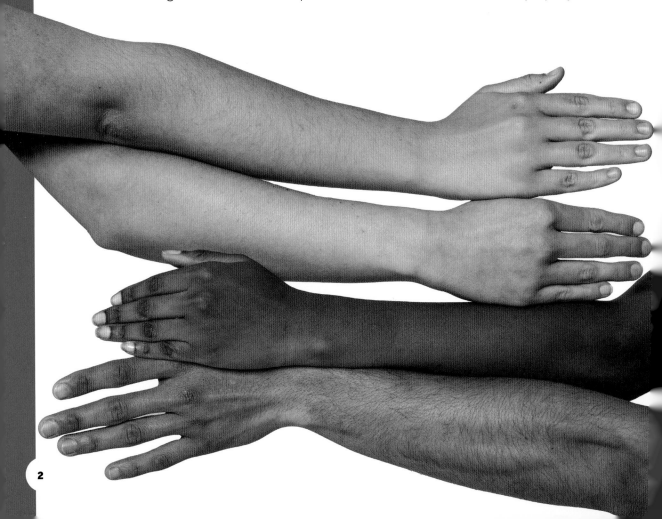

The skin has three layers: the epidermis, dermis, and hypodermis.

The epidermis is the top skin layer. This is where melanin is produced, which gives skin its color. While the epidermis is the thinnest layer, it's extremely tough, flexible, and waterproof. It's constantly shedding and replacing new skin cells, renewing itself every twenty-eight days or so throughout a person's entire life. That's why tanned skin eventually returns to its original paler color, and why many scars fade.

The dermis, the middle skin layer, is where 90 percent of your skin's thickness comes from. It's full of the body's sweat glands, sebaceous (oil) glands, nerve endings, and most of the body's hair follicles. (Skin pores are hair follicle openings.)

The bottom skin layer, the hypodermis (also called subcutaneous tissue), isn't exactly skin. In Greek, *hypoderm* means "beneath the skin." The hypodermis connects the top two layers of skin to the body's muscles and bones, regulates body temperature, and stores fat as energy reserves. The hypodermis also acts like bubble wrap for the inside of the body by protecting bones, organs, and muscles from injury.

> Skin is thickest on the soles of feet and palms of hands. Facial skin is much thinner and more prone to issues (like acne and chapped lips). The thinnest, most delicate skin is on the eyelids.

Skin Sweats!

Sweating is the body's air conditioner. Sweat is mostly water that exits your body through your skin's pores, where it sits on the skin's surface until it evaporates, causing a cooling effect. Your skin can constantly produce sweat as it automatically regulates your body temperature, but sometimes that sweat is in such small amounts that it's not even noticeable. When a lot of sweat exits the body, it can take time to fully evaporate, causing your skin to feel wet and slick.

Too Much Sweat!

Some people sweat more intensely than others, thanks to genetics. Almost everyone perspires when exercising, to help keep their body's temperature at its normal level. But many sweat more often—a lot more. Whether because of stress, anxiety, or hyperactive sweat glands, about 5 percent of people deal with hyperhidrosis, which is the medical term for superfluous sweating. Not only can hyperhidrosis make you feel uncomfortable, but pit stains, forehead beads, and slick palms can be noticeable and perhaps embarrassing.

Sometimes you're just born a super sweater, but occasionally, hyperhidrosis is a symptom of an underlying medical condition. So see your doctor if you suddenly start sweating more than usual.

A dermatologist is a type of doctor who treats skin conditions like excess sweating, acne, and more.

Not Enough Sweat

It's rare, but some people can't sweat enough, putting them at risk for heatstroke and other issues. This condition is called hypohidrosis. If you notice your ability to sweat decreasing, or you're not sweating after strenuous exercise or in the hot sun, see your doctor to find out if some of your sweat glands are blocked, if you're naturally missing some, or if you have this underlying medical condition.

Some people have a rare but harmless condition called chromhidrosis that causes their sweat to be colored pink, yellow, brown, or even blue.

Sweat Makes You Stink?

Sweat itself has no smell, but when it stays on your body for too long, odor arises. There are two types of sweat glands: eccrine and apocrine. Most sweat glands are eccrine glands, which produce a thin, watery sweat that has no aroma-producing ability but helps to cool down the body.

There are fewer apocrine sweat glands, but they pack a funky punch. Apocrine glands produce a thicker type of sweat full of fat and protein that bacteria love to break down into body odor.

Apocrine glands are concentrated in certain body parts, like the scalp, genitalia, and underarms, and aren't activated until puberty starts. That's why kids' armpits don't smell bad, because there's no fatty sweat for bacteria to convert into funk.

> Some scientists speculate that, in addition to causing body odor, apocrine gland secretions may also count as pheromones, which are testosterone-loaded substances that people emit (some more than others) that trigger a response from another person, whether a warning sign or sexual attraction.

Banishing Body Odor (Some of It, at Least)

Got B.O.? Oh no!

Everyone's body has an odor, and that's normal. It's not possible to get rid of all body odors permanently, but there are steps you can take to reduce them. To stave off stinkiness, ask yourself:

+ **Am I cleaning my body often and well?** The longer sweat and dirt stay on your skin, the more bacteria accumulate and the smellier you become. Bathing with soap and water daily (and, ideally, immediately after sweating extensively) gives bacteria less time to convert sweat into body odor. Bathing also helps to get rid of funk caused by other grime, like traces of urine and poop left on your body, and product buildup, such as deodorant layers. See page 10 for a head-to-toe body-washing game plan.

✦ **Are my clothes clean?** If your clothes don't pass the sniff test, neither will you, no matter how often you bathe. Wearing clothing (including underwear) without washing between wears can fuel your funk, as can certain clothing fabrics, especially synthetics. Polyester, rayon, and nylon tend to trap odor-causing bacteria, sometimes even after washing. Look for shirts and underwear made of more breathable, natural fabrics, such as cotton or linen.

✦ **What am I eating and drinking?** Some strong-smelling foods can cause body odor, too. Your body usually can't fully process the aroma of pungent foods like garlic and onions, so those odors are emitted through the skin's pores. Alcoholic drinks, Brussels sprouts, cauliflower, and red meat can also worsen body odor.

✦ **How do you feel?** People who are sick or very stressed sometimes give off a different odor. Occasionally, very smelly sweat is a medical condition called bromhidrosis, which means "foul-smelling sweat." People who suffer from bromhidrosis have bacteria on their bodies that produce particularly foul odors, especially when paired with hyperhidrosis (sweating too much; see page 4 for more). If ramping up your personal hygiene and eating more nutritious foods (like those on page 7) doesn't help, see your doctor.

Your ever-evolving hormones cause your body odor to change as you age, too, which is why babies, young children, teenagers, adults, and older people all smell different. So "old person smell" is really a thing!

Can These Foods Fix Your Funk?

While they don't work for everyone, and it can take a while to smell results, some foods have a reputation for reducing odor, including:

+ Chlorophyll-filled foods, like parsley, cilantro, spinach, chard, kale, and arugula

+ Citrus fruits, like grapefruit, oranges, and lemons

+ Certain spices, like fenugreek and cardamom. These have the opposite effect of garlic and onions, causing a sweet smell to emit from pores. Fenugreek, in particular, is known to cause "maple syrup sweat."

Body hair can be a flytrap for funk. If you're comfortable with the idea, trimming or removing body fuzz might help evict bacteria from their hairy homes, especially underneath your arms. Check out the hair-removal methods starting on page 61 for some tips.

Deodorant, Antiperspirant, or Body Sprays?

If you're trying to stop your underarms from smelling, consider an antiperspirant, deodorant, or combination of both. Antiperspirants block sweat glands, making you sweat less, but they don't stop odors. On the other hand, deodorants don't stop you from sweating, but they mask odor. Many people prefer to use both products, either in an all-in-one combination or separately. Some doctors suggest people use an anti-perspirant at night, right after bathing. Then, in the morning, adding a thin layer of deodorant on top of the antiperspirant is usually enough to keep you smelling fresh until your next shower.

There are many types of antiperspirants and deodorants, and every person's pits react differently to various ingredients, so explore multiple products (sticks, sprays, creams, and powders) until you find one that works for you. Products marked "clinical" tend to be stronger and perform better, although products marked "natural" work well for some people.

Whatever you choose to use, make sure to put it on freshly washed skin. Once the bacteria begin to break down the sweat, you won't be able to stop the stink fully, no matter how many layers of product you apply.

If, after experimenting, you find that an over-the-counter antiperspirant doesn't work wonders on your wetness, see your doctor. There are prescription options available that can be quite effective for axillary (underarm) hyperhidrosis. Sometimes, excessive sweating and odor are symptoms of a medical condition, such as an anxiety disorder, so checking in with your doctor can be a slick move.

> Body sprays have become very popular but are not a replacement for antiperspirants, as they only cover up funk, like deodorants and perfumes. Body sprays are also easy to overuse and have a very strong smell that might be offensive to others. So use just a spray or two, please!

Funky Feet

Even though there are no stink-stimulating apocrine glands on feet, there's a type of bacteria called brevibacterium that specifically thrives between sweaty toes. It's actually the same bacteria used to produce one of the smelliest cheeses in the world: Limburger, hence why sometimes stinky feet smell cheesy.

Are your feet bringing the funk? Ask yourself:

+ **Am I washing my feet well?** Scrub not just from heel to toe but also between each toe with soap and water. Make sure to remove any "toe jam," which develops when cheesy-smelling foot bacteria mixes with dead skin cells, fabric fibers from socks, and other body grime. If toe jam doesn't wash away easily, it might be a sign of something more serious, like a fungal infection—see page 44 for more on those possibilities.

+ **Am I drying my feet well?** After bathing, get your feet as dry as possible before putting on socks or shoes. Dry feet have less chance of becoming smelly than damp feet. Moist feet are also perfect places for yeast or fungal infections, like athlete's foot, to fester. If your feet are damp because of sweat, consider using over-the-counter products sold specifically for foot sweat, or you can also use the same antiperspirant and deodorant you use for underarms on your feet.

+ **Do my shoes stink?** Foul feet could be caused by your footwear. It's often a vicious cycle of smells that starts with foot funk—especially if you don't wear socks with your shoes. Stink from your feet can seep into the fabric of the inner lining and intensify in the dark, moist environment.

Aside from keeping feet as clean and dry as possible, here are some additional tips to prevent smelly shoes:

+ When it's warm enough or you're not exercising, wear breathable shoes, like open-toed shoes or rubber clogs.

+ Wear socks, as having a barrier between your feet and your footwear can help. Change socks multiple times per day (like after exercising) if your feet sweat a lot.

+ Insert removable, washable insoles inside your shoes.

+ Rotate your shoe collection, giving each pair at least a day or two to air out.

+ Spray the insides of your shoes with either vinegar (which neutralizes odors) or a shoe odor spray that you can buy at the drugstore. Let dry before re-wearing.

+ Try machine washing your shoes, if possible. Adding vinegar to the rinse cycle and letting them air-dry in direct sunlight might help with odor.

The Bathing Blueprint

How to wash your body might seem like a topic better suited for a kids' manual, but trust that *many* a person makes it to their twenties (and beyond) without knowing they're supposed to lather up their legs, crack into crevices, and de-gunk their genitalia on a daily basis. This doesn't have to be you!

Just as important as bathing *often* enough (every single day!) is bathing *properly*.

Do you hop out of the bath or shower and still seem sort of stinky? If so, some of your crannies might still be covered in bad-smell-making bacteria.

To truly banish body odor, you—yes, you—might need to read this blueprint that shows how to give your body a solid scrub-down in the shower.

First, gather what you need, including:

✦ **Body wash or bar soap.** Products that are dye-free and fragrance-free or products formulated for sensitive skin can help avoid allergic reactions and irritation.

✦ **A clean skin scrubber.** While using your hands is better than nothing, gently scrubbing your body with a washcloth, shower mitt, loofah, or sponge helps remove more bacteria, dead skin cells, and dirt.

✦ **A fresh towel.** Ideally, you should use a clean towel every time you bathe, as bacteria breeds on damp, used towels, meaning you'll just be spreading old, musty germs all over your freshly washed body. If you can't use a clean towel every time, make sure to hang it up between uses to let it air out.

✦ **Deodorant and/or antiperspirant.** (Turn to page 7 to learn the difference.) You'll use this after you bathe on your freshly washed and dried body.

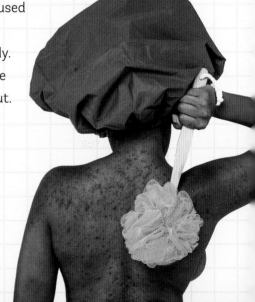

- **A toothbrush and toothpaste.** Twice-daily brushing is important, and it might be easiest to incorporate one toothbrushing after, during, or before bathing to create a routine.

- **A shower chair, safety rail, or other needed safety accessory.** If standing for long periods or getting out of the tub is difficult or impossible, make sure your bathroom is equipped with the items you need to scrub your body safely.

> Between 5 and 10 percent of Americans under the age of twenty-two are living with some type of disability that may impact their ability to independently groom and bathe. If you relate to this statistic, as your body changes, you might find your cleaning needs changing, too. Know that it's okay (and a great idea that should have zero shame attached) to ask for more assistance, such as getting help bathing more often or cleaning more thoroughly—or more gently—in certain crevices (such as the folds of your genitalia) so you can achieve the level of cleanliness and comfort that you deserve.

NOW FOR THE BATHING BASICS:

- **Start at the top and work your way down.** Your body tends to get dirtier as you move down from your head to your feet.

- **Hair washing is optional (but don't forget your scalp when you do).** Your hair (and the scalp it grows from) can become stinky and grimy pretty quickly, especially during puberty. But depending upon your hairstyle or your hair type, you might not wash your hair every day. That's perfectly normal and healthy—there's a reason millions of shower caps are sold every year. However, when you do wash and condition your hair, whether it's in the shower or at a sink, don't forget to scrub your scalp with either your fingers or a special silicone scalp scrubber to remove dandruff and product buildup.

✦ **Face and teeth time is necessary.** Facial skin is extremely delicate and sensitive, so you'll likely need different cleansing products, just like you need toothpaste and a toothbrush. You might like to wash your face or brush your teeth while bathing, or you may have a routine that you prefer to do separately—whatever works for you and your skin. See page 21 for face washing suggestions.

While a steaming hot shower can feel amazing, it can also be drying to the skin (see page 15 for more on dry skin). Lukewarm water is best for bathing, especially for people with sensitive skin.

TIME FOR THE BATHING BLUEPRINT!

STEP 1

Neck. Wet your sponge, washcloth, or other skin scrubber and apply your favorite body wash or bar soap. Then, with gentle circular motions, start scrubbing your entire neck and behind your ears to get rid of any grime. Use your fingers to clean the folds of your ears, too—these tiny crevices can get funky fast!

STEP 2

Arms. Starting at your fingernails, work your washcloth up and around each arm, making sure to get soap lather on everything, including both elbows. Spend more time and use more pressure to scrub your armpits well.

STEP 3

Chest. Now get to work on your chest. If you have large breasts, be sure to lift up each one individually and gently scrub your underboob well—bacteria love to colonize in this area.

STEP 4

Stomach. Next, move down and wash your stomach, being sure to get into your belly button (it can help to use a finger with a little soap to gently dig out any dirt in there).

STEP 5

Back. Then start scrubbing your entire back, making sure to hit the hard-to-reach center. A loofah on a stick can come in handy.

STEP 6

Genitalia. Your genitalia require a little extra time and attention, as the hair and folds love to hold on to and hide bacteria and grime. Rinse and re-soap your scrubber and use it to gently scrub your inner thighs and any parts covered in pubic hair. Then use your fingers and water (no soap) to clean your penis and scrotum or your vulva, ridding the area of any gunk, such as the totally normal but sometimes stinky cottage-cheese-like substance called smegma (see page 126 for more on smegma).

People with vaginas should be sure to use their fingers to individually clean the labial folds (see page 143 for more on the labia). Be careful not to get any soap in your vaginal canal, unless your doctor says otherwise, as soap can irritate and cause pain in this sensitive area.

People with uncircumcised penises should also avoid getting soap underneath their foreskin. Always gently pull back the foreskin and clean the glans (penis head) with water and your fingers.

STEP 7

Butt crack. Now, rinse and re-soap your scrubber and start lathering your rear. Don't skip washing your anus (butthole) directly. To really get in there, lift your legs one at a time (maybe using the edge of the tub for balance) and scrub-a-dub-dub, making sure to re-soap and rinse with clean water often.

STEP 8

Legs. Thoroughly rinse and re-soap your washcloth or sponge (or get a new one if your butt was especially dirty), and scrub down and around each one of your legs. It's not enough to just let water run down your legs; they need to be directly washed.

STEP 9

Feet. Rinse and re-soap your scrubber and get between each of your toes. Scrub your heels and soles well, too.

Rinse everything. Set aside your scrubber and rinse off all leftover suds, getting into every nook and cranny. Spread your bottom cheeks and, if you have them, the folds of your labia. Retract your foreskin, if you have it, so you can easily rinse there with water, too. Be thorough, from your armpits to your ankles, as soap that remains on the body post-bathing can be drying and irritating to the skin.

Dry everywhere. Use your towel to get into all the crevices you just cleaned, drying them as best you can. Because dry bodies stay stink-free for longer, consider using a hair dryer on a cool setting, especially under your breasts, behind your scrotum, and between your toes.

Apply products. Once you've toweled off, apply your deodorant, antiperspirant, and any other products, like foot powder and body lotion.

When Bathing Feels Impossible

Depression, autism, attention-deficit/hyperactivity disorder (ADHD), and other conditions can make it feel difficult—even impossible—to bathe once a day or even once per week. If you relate to this, try taking things in steps. First, commit to brushing your teeth at least once a day, because dirty teeth tend to cause more permanent damage than dirty skin. Then try to add genital and underarm washing to your can-do list, as those tend to be the smelliest, stickiest body bits. Sometimes, if you can't bring yourself to get into the shower or tub, putting a package of body wipes in the bathroom and committing to washing your crevices when you use the toilet is absolutely better than nothing; just don't flush them afterward, no matter what the packaging says, or you might soon have a plumbing problem.

Dry Skin? Save Your Skin Barrier!

Most people deal with dry skin at some point in their lives, especially during colder months. Dry skin starts on the top layer, the epidermis, which is essentially a bunch of cells glued together by an oily layer made up of fat and cholesterol, known as lipids. The mixture of lipids and cells creates a waterproof skin barrier that helps your skin retain moisture.

Sometimes your body doesn't produce enough lipids for your cells to form a waterproof barrier. This leads to moisture loss, which causes dry skin. While dry skin can feel uncomfortable, by itself it isn't threatening to health. However, dry skin often feels itchy and tightly stretched, which makes you want to scratch it. But scratching can easily damage dry skin, worsening scales and cracks until they become bleeding wounds, infections, and other skin disorders.

Here are some lipid-saving techniques to help keep skin soft and improve its appearance:

+ **Cleanse with care.** Harsh scrubbing, hot water, and excess soap dry the skin, which allows moisture to escape. During your daily bath or shower, use lukewarm water and less soap than usual to gently wash, not polish, your skin. The soap you use should be moisturizing, and on the parts of your body suffering from dry skin, avoid products containing harsh ingredients, such as antibacterial soaps.

+ **Exfoliate.** While you don't want to scrub your body harshly every day, a weekly body exfoliation is an excellent way to remove the buildup of dead skin cells, which can tinge skin gray or white—some people refer to this coloration as looking "ashy." Exfoliation also stimulates new skin cell growth and improves the texture of your skin. While you can pick up body scrubs at any store, you can also easily make your own. Blend together 6 tablespoons of oatmeal, 4 tablespoons of water, and 2 tablespoons of honey. Add a little bit more water if the mixture needs to be thinned to spread. While standing in the shower, massage this concoction all over your body. Wait two minutes before using a washcloth to scrub it off and see if it makes a difference. If your skin isn't especially sensitive, add 1 to 2 tablespoons of sugar for additional exfoliating power. When you're done, don't forget to clean any oatmeal bits out of the tub and discard any remaining mixture.

+ **Moisturize.** It's almost impossible to over-moisturize your skin! If you suffer from dry skin, slather on an emollient, ideally once a day right after you bathe. Emollients are ingredients that act like lipids, helping create a moisture-conserving, waterproof skin barrier by filling in cracks and sealing the skin. Emollients include cocoa butter, coconut oil, paraffin, olive oil, beeswax, and lanolin. If you're not allergic, coconut oil can be a good choice as an allover moisturizer, as it's an emollient and naturally antibacterial. You can even use coconut oil on your genitalia (vulvas and penises can sometimes dry out, too).

+ **Practice healthy habits.** Eating enough "good" fats like coconut oil, nuts, seeds, and foods with plenty of omega-3s can help improve dry skin. If you smoke or visit tanning salons, you may be lowering your life span, drying your skin, and causing premature wrinkling at the same time. So, stop! (See page 205 for more on healthy self-care habits.)

+ **Drink water.** While water intake alone isn't enough to eliminate dry skin, drinking water is crucial to preventing dehydration, which worsens dry skin.

The medical term for extremely dry skin is "xerosis." Signs include rough spots, rashes, scales, cracks, and cuts either all over your body or concentrated in specific areas, like your elbows or knees.

Chapped Lips

Lips are skin, too! Lips help us eat, speak, and sense temperature. Without lips, people couldn't kiss or whistle. And your lip imprint (what's left behind if you put on lipstick and kiss a piece of paper) is as unique and one-of-a-kind as your fingerprint.

When lips get overly dry, they can become chapped. There are many causes for chapped lips: dehydration, frequent licking, certain medications, sun exposure, and dry or cold weather can all be culprits.

Fortunately, there are some easy ways to heal chapped lips. First, slather them with a thick layer of moisturizer that is safe for lips, like coconut oil, beeswax, or cocoa butter. Consider one with an SPF if you spend a lot of time outdoors, as sun damage can cause chapped lips, too. Continue to reapply throughout the day and before you go to sleep. Next, you can exfoliate dead lip skin by gently rubbing a wet washcloth over your lips before reapplying your moisturizer of choice. Finally, drinking more water can work wonders in preventing and healing chapped lips.

Most importantly—stop licking or sucking on your lips! Even though it makes chapped lips feel better for a couple of seconds, your saliva is designed to help digest food, not to hydrate lips, so when you lick, it irritates the skin around your mouth and can make the situation worse, even causing a condition like angular cheilitis, where mouth corners can become painful and inflamed.

See your doctor if your chapped lips don't heal with these suggestions, as you may need a stronger moisturizer or a different treatment plan.

What's on My Upper Lip?

Scary-looking lip lumps can start with a simple tingle on or around your mouth . . . but before you know it, there's an enormous, painful, ugly, and possibly oozy sore front and center on your face! Random spots and sores like this are probably a sign that you're infected with a strain of herpes simplex virus (HSV). But you're not alone—most people have HSV, which can be a sexually transmitted infection (STI), but some strains also affect people who've never had sex.

Often the erupting skin spot is called a cold sore or fever blister and is caused by herpes simplex virus 1 (HSV-1). HSV-1 is not sexually transmitted but instead spreads by sharing personal items like towels and cups, and by kissing. It's even possible to have gotten HSV-1 as a baby from being kissed by an infected adult.

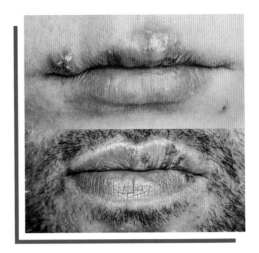

If you've had oral sex or sexual intercourse and a sore shows up, it could be a strain of herpes that's an STI, likely herpes simplex virus 2 (HSV-2). HSV-2 often shows up on the genitals, but it can pop up on the face, too. See page 127 for more on sexually transmitted herpes.

HSV-1 and HSV-2 often look the same, and both can make surprise appearances on the face or genitalia, so don't stress yourself out trying to self-diagnose.

Since all types of herpes are contagious, avoid any sort of skin-to-skin contact during an outbreak. And if you see a sore on your sexual partner, ask for a rain check on romantic actions and suggest they see their doctor.

It's much easier to diagnose herpes when sores are visible, so see your doctor when you're dealing with an outbreak. Whether it's a cold sore or an STI, they may be able to help speed up the healing process and can also, if needed, test you for other possible STIs (see page 185 for more).

> Remember: we're all different, and as you can see from the two pictures on this page, what symptoms of something like herpes (or ringworm or cystic acne, or other issues discussed later in this manual) look like on your skin may not be exactly the same as what's represented by the pictures in this manual . . . or even anywhere on the Internet. And that's totally expected, normal, and okay! If you have a concern you can't figure out, see your doctor.

All Kinds of Acne

Dealing with acne? Pore you!

"Acne" is the medical term for when your skin's pores (also known as hair follicles) are clogged by oil, sweat, bacteria, and dead cells, causing pimples and many other types of spots to appear on your face and body.

Because puberty messes with hormones and triggers extra oil production, more than 4 out of every 5 people have to put up with acne between the ages of twelve and twenty-four, and often in the years beyond.

There are a number of different types of acne. In order of severity (least to worst), they include:

+ **Whiteheads.** Blocked hair follicles that appear to have white "heads" because they stay beneath the skin's surface. Whiteheads clear up faster than other types of pimples.

+ **Blackheads.** Whiteheads that rise to the surface of the skin and open up, turning black when the oil inside the pimple mixes with oxygen in the air.

+ **Papules.** Small, solid bumps that are inflamed and feel sore when touched.

+ **Pustules.** What most people think of when they hear the word "pimples." They have white or yellow pus-filled "heads" and can appear red around the base.

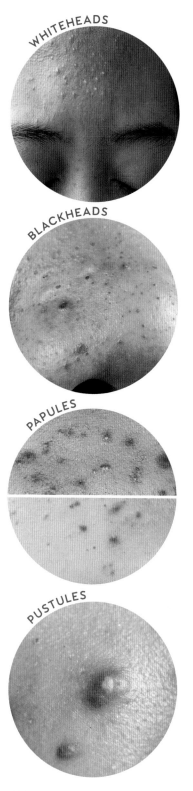

WHITEHEADS

BLACKHEADS

PAPULES

PUSTULES

- ✦ **Nodules.** Nodules are larger, hard, and sometimes painful bumps embedded deeply in the skin. Nodules can last for months and often cause scarring.

- ✦ **Cysts.** Nodules are often paired with cysts, which are sacs filled with fluid, pus, or semisolid material under the skin that can become inflamed and infected (and can multiply!). Also called cystic acne, cysts can be very painful and sometimes cause extreme scarring.

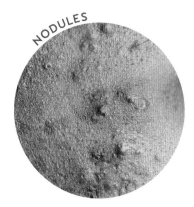

NODULES

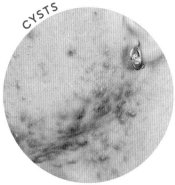

CYSTS

If you're dealing with the more severe forms of acne, which are papules, pustules, nodules, and cysts, consider seeing a doctor, especially one who specializes in skin (a dermatologist). They can help you figure out what's going on with your face and possibly reduce spots and minimize scarring with treatment and medication.

It's common to use the terms "skin pores" and "hair follicles" interchangeably when talking about skin care. Skin pores are just the openings to hair follicles.

Got Pimples? Stop the Pop!

Yes, it may feel great to squeeze a pimple, but it's never worth it. For starters, it's impossible to completely empty the pore of pus, so your pimple will eventually come back in exactly the same spot—this has probably already happened to you, right? Even if, somehow, you get out most of the pus, you'll likely end up spreading more pimple-causing bacteria during the popping process, which could create even more pimples!

Popping pimples can also lead to acne scars, but sometimes even pimples that you ignore can leave behind dark spots. Are you battling blemishes and scars from past bouts with acne on your face and body? The answer is probably "yes," but don't worry. As your skin renews itself, many of your skin stains will disappear over time. Keep reading for additional suggestions on how to avoid long-term acne scars and other forms of hyperpigmentation (page 38).

Skin Care Suggestions

Remember, acne is the most common skin disorder in America, but dealing with it can still feel isolating, embarrassing, and overwhelming. Try not to take your acne personally, as no matter how (literally) painful it is, it tends to be just a rite of passage that most people go through.

Teen acne usually improves over time, after your body's oil production slows down in your late teens or early twenties. Regardless of your age, there are ways to manage and improve acne, including:

- **Clean your skin with care.** While a clean face can't prevent all pimples, it does help to remove gunk and grime that can clog and infect hair follicles. Acne-prone people can look for cleansers that contain ingredients designed to shut down zit factories, like salicylic acid. To minimize skin damage, avoid harsh scrubbing with intense exfoliants (which can make things worse), and always pat your face dry with a clean towel—vigorous rubbing can irritate the skin. For body washing tips, see page 10.

- **Clean your stuff often.** Sleeping on a dirty pillow, wearing dirty clothes, and using dirty reusable items like washcloths, applicator sponges, and makeup brushes can cause breakouts. Frequently wash anything that comes in contact with your skin to help remove breakout-causing bacteria.

- **Treat the worst spots.** Sometimes over-the-counter acne medicine can help, but to avoid making your skin worse, test the product out on a small area before slathering it all over, and read package directions before use. Always be careful not to use harsh products near delicate skin like your eyelids and genitalia.

+ **Check personal care products.** If you're using hair oil, gel, or spray that might be dripping onto your forehead or cheeks, they might be a cause of some of your pimples.

+ **Hats off.** If you often wear a helmet, hat, or headband and you notice a bunch of brow bumps, the constant friction of sweaty, dirty, bacteria-covered material against your forehead is the likely culprit. Similarly, jewelry can cause acne and other skin irritation.

+ **Relax.** Stress makes acne worse. (Stress makes everything worse.) See page 205 for a self-care checklist that might help you manage your feelings about your skin (and life in general).

+ **Loosen up.** Tight clothing can create the perfect opportunity for body-acne-causing bacteria to breed by trapping dirt and sweat, so peel off your stinky sweats ASAP after exercising.

+ **Be patient.** Spots can show up overnight, but getting them to disappear can take weeks, and the dark spots and scars they leave behind can last even longer. You can pass the time and help your skin heal by staying hydrated, getting enough sleep, and taking care of yourself in other ways.

See your doctor (especially a dermatologist) if your skin-care routine isn't putting a dent in the number of dots on your face. They can examine your skin, give more tailored advice, and, if necessary, prescribe medication.

Makeup itself does not usually cause breakouts, but you can make your pimple problem worse if you put makeup on a dirty face or leave it on overnight. Always apply makeup to a clean face and wash it all off before bed!

Skin-Picking Disorder

Most of us pop a pimple or pick at a scab every now and then, even though we know better. But around 1 out of every 50 people has a skin-picking disorder where the need to pick, pop, or scratch at their face or body is compulsive, meaning it's very hard to stop, even when it causes severe pain and scarring. People with this skin-picking disorder, called dermatillomania, often also have trichotillomania, or hair-pulling disorder (see page 66 for more). Like with hair pulling, compulsive skin picking is a physical symptom of a mental health issue, and it's important to seek professional help for support and to develop strategies and coping mechanisms to stop. See page 198 for types of therapists to consider.

Body Acne

Since hair follicles are found almost everywhere on your body, acne can crop up almost anywhere, too, from your neck to your butt to even your genitalia. Sometimes body acne is more uncomfortable and difficult to deal with than facial acne, because it's often in constant contact with clothes, which can cause friction (and possibly folliculitis; see page 24). Treatment options for body

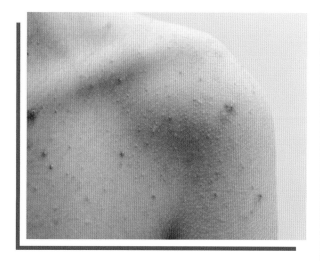

acne are generally the same as for facial acne, though products marketed for body acne are often stronger, as body skin tends to be less fragile than facial skin. Your doctor can help you get a handle on body acne, too.

Follicu-what?

Your face and body bumps might not be acne but folliculitis, an often pus-filled and painful bumpy rash that looks and feels a lot like acne pimples. Unlike acne, folliculitis tends to occur mostly in damaged hair follicles, as the damage makes it easier for pores/follicles to become infected by bacteria and other germs, causing a concentrated crop of bumps. Hair follicle damage often happens from friction (like from a bra strap, jockstrap, or thigh chafing), frequent skin rubbing (like from a headband or mask), and shaving (especially with a dull razor).

There are many different types of folliculitis, including:

✦ **Infected ingrown hairs/razor bumps.** An infection from a hair curling back into the follicle. Often, razor bumps start with damage from shaving (razor burn), but any type of hair-removal technique can cause ingrown hairs, and any ingrown hairs can become infected and turn into folliculitis. (See page 65 for more on ingrown hairs.)

✦ **Genital folliculitis.** Thigh and pubic hair follicle infection from friction, usually by clothing, sex, or hair removal.

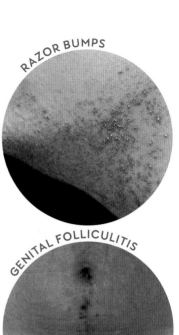

RAZOR BUMPS

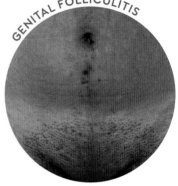

GENITAL FOLLICULITIS

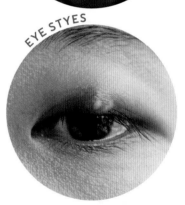

EYE STYES

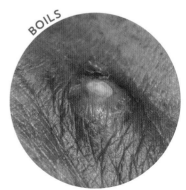

BOILS

- **Eye styes.** When an eyelash follicle becomes infected, a stye is formed.

- **Boils.** Follicle infections from fungi or bacteria. Cystic acne and ingrown hairs can sometimes turn into a boil, which is large, pus-filled, and often painful. Boils are also called furuncles, and when skin is so infected that there are a bunch of boils in one location, it's called a carbuncle.

Since folliculitis is so similar to acne, it can be difficult to detect a difference. Often there are signs of infection, like a red ring around each swollen folliculitis bump. But acne can become infected and swollen, too. Fortunately, treatment is the same: do not pop—and keep the area very clean. More often than not, folliculitis will go away by itself, but see your doctor for possible treatment if, after a week or so of careful observation, the bumps:

- Become larger, redder, more tender, or smellier

- Are accompanied by fever, pain, itching, burning, or odor

There's also "hot tub" folliculitis, which looks identical to many other types of folliculitis but happens when a person's follicles are infected by a specific type of bacteria generally found only in hot tubs.

Goose Bumps

Goose bumps are another type of hair follicle bump, but not one caused by irritation or infection. When your body is cold, tiny muscles involuntarily contract, raising your hair follicles and creating goose bumps in the process of conserving and generating heat. Goose bumps also form when you're scared or excited—if an emotion "gives you chills," likely it also gives you goose bumps. Eventually, when you calm down or warm up, the muscles relax and the goose bumps disappear.

Freckles

No one is born with freckles, but some of us are born with the freckle gene. People with the freckle gene have extra melanin in some of their skin cells that, when exposed to UV rays in sunlight, darken and become freckles. That's why babies aren't born with freckles—because they haven't been in the sun yet. Individual freckles can be almost too small to see or as large as a remote control button—or they can be clumped together and may look even larger. Some people have seasonal freckles that show up only in the summer, while others keep theirs year-round. Using sunscreen can sometimes help stop freckles from sprouting, if desired.

Warts

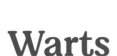

Warts are rough-surfaced, cauliflower-like raised bumps that are caused by a harmless strain of human papillomavirus, known as HPV (not the genital type). Warts are very contagious and can spread through skin-to-skin contact.

Most warts disappear on their own within two years, but they can also be treated or removed by a doctor or with over-the-counter medication. Warts can be found all over the body, and some have specific names, like plantar (foot) warts. They are not cancerous, though some skin cancers look like warts. Genital warts often can look identical to "regular" warts, too. See page 127 for more on genital warts.

Molluscum Contagiosum

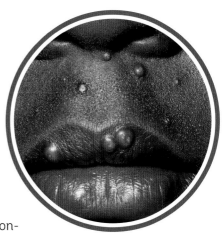

Another common infection that causes wart-like lesions is molluscum contagiosum. This virus is easily transmitted through skin-to-skin contact and usually clears up on its own. Your doctor can determine if the lesions, which can appear anywhere on your body (including your genitals), are caused by HPV or the virus that causes molluscum contagiosum, and can treat them accordingly.

Skin Tags

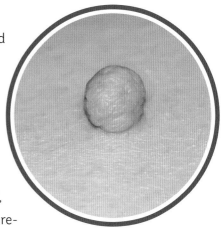

Skin tags look like little nubs or flaps on your body and are the same color as the rest of your skin. They aren't contagious and are usually from friction (like the collar of your shirt rubbing up against your neck), which causes the top layer of your skin in that area to grow extra cells. If you'd like to get your skin tags removed, don't try to DIY. Even though they look like they would be easy to snip off, there is a risk of extreme bleeding and infection if removed improperly. See your doctor.

Moles

Whereas freckles are always flat, moles are clusters of pigmented cells that can be raised or flat. Moles can also sprout hair. Some moles are hereditary, and when they're present at birth, moles are a type of permanent birthmark, but they can pop up on your skin at any time in life. While all body spots should be checked frequently for any changes, moles should be closely monitored to watch for possible skin cancers, especially if they're new. See the next section for how to check your skin spots.

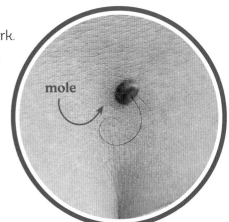

Is It Skin Cancer?

Whether you're born with a bunch of pigmented spots on your skin or they crop up unexpectedly, it's important to try to keep up with any changes in size, shape, color, and texture and to keep your doctor posted—especially if cancer runs in your family, as many pigmented body spots can become cancerous.

   Experts suggest checking your entire body (including nail beds, palms of hands, and soles of feet) at least once a month and examine any skin spots using the skin cancer detection ABCDEs:

- **A = asymmetry.** Is your skin growth not symmetrical (the fancy word for perfectly round)?

- **B = border irregularities.** Is the border of your skin growth ragged and uneven?

- **C = color changing.** Is the skin growth darker than your other growths, two-toned, or tan one month and dark brown another?

- **D = diameter.** Is the skin growth the size of a pencil eraser or larger?

- **E = evolving.** Has something changed recently, like is the area larger, painful, or bleeding?

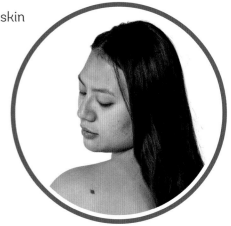

If it's too much to write everything down, taking pictures every few months and comparing them can be helpful, too.

See your doctor IMMEDIATELY if you answer "yes" to any of the ABCDEs, as skin cancer among young adults is on the rise but is very treatable when caught early.

)   Sunscreen also provides additional benefits, like wrinkle prevention.   )

Dark Skin Needs Skin Cancer Screenings and Sunscreen, Too!

People of color aren't off the hook when it comes to sunscreen and skin checkups—no one is immune to skin cancer caused by the sun, and while people with darker skin may be less prone to skin cancers caused by UV rays than people with lighter skin, it's not impossible.

Plus, skin checkups are important because skin cancer often isn't related to sun exposure, so cancerous spots can present differently, such as on the palms and soles of feet and under nail beds (see page 44 for more on nail cancer). So be sure to check those body parts, too, and see a dermatologist if any strange spots crop up.

Lips need sunscreen, too—no one wants a sunburned smoocher! Either rub your regular sunscreen on them as part of your personal care routine or purchase one of the many lip balms formulated with an SPF of at least 30.

Preventing Skin Cancer

While people with very fair hair and skin, several moles, close relatives with moles, or a family history of skin cancer are at higher risk of getting skin cancer, anyone can be diagnosed, so it's important to protect yourself. Follow these suggestions to best avoid carcinogenic (cancer-causing) UV rays:

- ✦ **Slather on sunscreen.** Everyone knows to use sunscreen, but do you know what *kind* you should use? Sunscreen is sold in different SPFs, which measures how well it can protect against UV rays. The higher the SPF, the more UV rays it claims to block. A sunscreen of at least 30 SPF is recommended for everyone, regardless of climate or skin type. The sun still emits harmful UV rays in colder weather, so try to wear sunscreen all year long. Make sure to get it on every exposed body part—from behind the ears to between your nostrils to the middle of your back. Many brands have separate sunscreen formulations for the face and body, with body versions tending to be thicker and more visible on the skin, and face versions more invisible. If appearance doesn't matter as much to you, and you don't have especially sensitive skin, you can use body sunscreen on your face. You can also use face sunscreen on your body, but that could get very costly fast.

- ✦ **Cover up with clothing.** Covering up much of your body is a great way to block UV rays, especially if you can buy or borrow Ultraviolet Protection Factor (UPF) clothing, which is made to block UV rays. When possible, wear sunglasses and a wide-brimmed hat to protect your head, face, and eyes.

- ✦ **Stay in the shade.** Avoiding direct sunlight helps to minimize contact with penetrating UV rays. Bringing an umbrella or tent to the beach can help you safely have fun in the sun.

- ✦ **Check vitamin D levels.** Vitamin D has many benefits, one of which is the prevention of some types of skin cancer, which is ironic considering it is naturally absorbed from the sun. But many people are deficient, especially people with darker skin, who have difficulty absorbing vitamin D from the sun. At your next physical, ask your doctor to order a blood test to check your levels, and consider supplements if the results come back low.

Sun protection is about more than just cancer prevention. Limiting sun exposure also keeps your skin smooth and sunburn free.

The UV lights used to cure gel manicures have been linked to numerous cases of skin cancers on the hand. If you love getting gel manicures, wear sunscreen on your hands during the curing of the polish or consider switching to a nail-painting option that doesn't involve UV rays.

Butt and Thigh Lumps

Cellulite isn't considered a medical concern, but when it unexpectedly shows up and rear-ends us, the resulting lumps and bumps can cause damage to self-esteem. Cellulite happens when body fat pushes up against skin's connective tissue, which creates visible surface lumps. These body ripples are commonly found on stomachs, hips, thighs, and butts. Though cellulite can happen to anyone, regardless of weight or body type, the amount you have has been linked to age, genetics, weight, and a person's eating and exercise habits. So if one or both of your biological parents have dimpled derrieres or if you're not eating healthfully or exercising, you might be more likely to have cellulite. Since testosterone prevents the development of cellulite, only around 10 percent of people born with penises tend to have it—compared to over 80 percent of people born with vaginas.

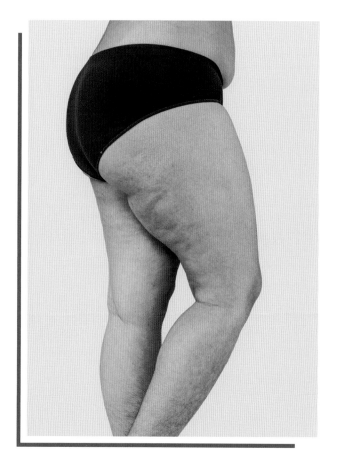

No pill, potion, or lotion has been proven to cure stretch marks or cellulite. What can help is drinking plenty of water and keeping your skin moisturized, as hydrated skin minimizes the appearance of stretch marks and cellulite. Also, while exercising won't get rid of cellulite or stretch marks, lifting weights and doing cardiovascular work tightens and tones areas that are cellulite- and stretch-mark-prone.

Stretch Marks

Sometimes your body grows so quickly, either in height or weight, that your skin can't keep up the pace—especially during puberty. As your skin stretches quickly to accommodate the extra inches, the connective fibers break, creating the striped scars we call stretch marks.

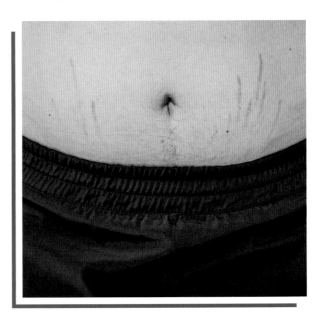

Although stretch marks can be found anywhere, they show up most frequently on chests, breasts, stomachs, arms, hips, butts, and thighs. Some people, such as those with drier skin or a history of stretch marks in their family, are more prone than others. Usually stretch marks fade gradually over time, from darker, more obvious colors to less noticeable lines, or they disappear altogether.

Stretch marks are a kind of scar!

Scars: The Skin's Battle Wounds

Skin works hard to protect your body, and sometimes it gets injured in the process. When this happens, skin immediately starts to repair itself. First, blood rushes to the injury, which then quickly clots and coagulates into a protective scab. Depending upon how large and deep the injury is, as well as how often you pick at your scab (we've all done it), your skin often leaves behind some sort of scar as it heals. Not all skin injuries leave scars, but many do. Common skin injuries that can cause scarring include:

+ Accidental wounds, like scratches, cuts, punctures, or burns

+ Purposeful wounds, like tattoos, piercings, or surgery

+ Acne (especially if you squeeze or pop pimples)

+ Illnesses or infections (especially ones that cause sores or rashes)

Superficial scars, meaning just the epidermis (the top layer of skin) was scraped or punctured, eventually fade as your skin sheds. When wounds go into deeper layers of skin (dermis) that don't constantly have cells that die and replace themselves, scars last much longer and are more obvious. That's why tattoos are permanent; the wounds the tattoo needle makes puncture deep into the skin, to the layers that don't renew themselves.

When possible, instead of letting a scab dry out and form a hard crust, keep it moist by covering it with ointment and a clean bandage every day; this can help prevent infection and scarring. If you're trying to improve the appearance of an existing scar, staying hydrated and moisturized goes a long way. Gentle exfoliation can also speed up the skin-renewal process (see page 15 for more). If your scar is serious enough, your doctor may have solutions to minimize its appearance.

But remember: a scar is proof of strength and survival, so perhaps embracing it as part of yourself is worth a shot!

Keloids

Some scars are thicker and more prominent than others. That's because some bodies, especially ones with more melanin, get overenthusiastic about the wound-healing process and, instead of a basic scar, form mounds of itchy, thick, lumpy, and puckered tissue called keloids. Keloids can pop up around any type of wound—including piercings and tattoos.

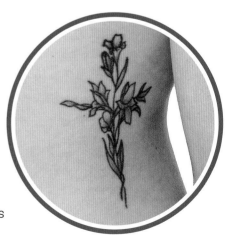

Until a keloid forms on your body, there's no way to know if your skin is keloid-prone. Since it can be genetic, if someone in your biological family has a keloid, consider rethinking your piercing or tattoo. Sometimes it can help to see your doctor beforehand, as they may be able to offer medication to help stave off these intense scars.

> Scars are usually from injuries that happen to us, but sometimes we hurt ourselves on purpose. See page 203 for more information on mental health and self-harm.

Piercings and Tattoos

Tattoos and piercings can be incredible forms of self-expression—when done properly by a professional. While a leg tattoo or lip piercing might seem fun and carefree, many body modifications carry a lifetime of responsibility, and it's very easy for them to become infected, as it can take from weeks (tattoos) to a year (some piercings) for them to fully heal. That's why it's extremely important to work with piercers and tattoo artists who are thoughtful, licensed (when possible), and hygienic.

Before you get pierced or tattooed, be sure to watch the professional work on someone else and note their cleanliness. If they don't practice perfect sterilization (always using new needles and having clean, gloved hands), and if they don't behave in a professional manner, find someone else to do the work. Some medical and piercing organizations suggest avoiding piercing guns altogether, saying they are impossible to fully sterilize and that they carry a higher risk of rejected piercings and serious infections.

And never try to DIY a body modification! Without a true professional working on your body, you run a much higher risk of getting a serious infection or injury; even nerve damage is possible.

> Before you get a body modification, make sure you're really ready, because regret is real and very common. Closed piercings can leave behind scars, and once inked in, tattoos can be expensive and difficult—sometimes impossible—to remove.

After you're pierced or tattooed, aftercare at home is crucial, as even a perfectly done body modification can become infected if you don't take care of the wound properly. Your piercer or tattoo artist should give you information on how to best take care of the wound—it's a good idea to ask for aftercare advice up front, and if they don't seem to take aftercare seriously, you might want to find another professional.

Signs your tattoo or piercing might be infected include:

✦ Soreness

✦ Redness

✦ Swelling

✦ Pain

✦ Funny smells

✦ Dripping pus

✦ Fever and/or chills

If you experience any of these symptoms, see your doctor ASAP.

Certain piercings can carry even *more* responsibility. For example, genitalia piercings may compromise condom use. Mouth piercings can be especially troublesome because you could accidentally swallow your jewelry, injure salivary glands, lose your sense of taste, or experience speech impediments, chipped teeth, uncontrolled drooling, nerve disorders, and even heart disease.

While you might not want to see your doctor for an infected tattoo or piercing because you fear they might judge you or tell you to take a piercing out, unfortunately, an infected tattoo or piercing has a high chance of worsening without treatment, and you could develop serious health problems or in rare cases even die. It's always a better idea to lose your piercing instead of your tongue, so see your doctor if something's wrong!

Depending on your age, you might want to settle for a fake tattoo or piercing for now. Many states have laws against some types of body modification for people under eighteen, regardless of parental consent. The government isn't trying to ruin your fun; the laws are there to protect you from health concerns as well as disfigurement. For example, if you pierce or tattoo the skin of an area that's still growing, there's a chance that your tattoo or piercing might stretch, causing it to look bad.

What Is Hypopigmentation?

Most people can find natural color variations all over their skin, thanks to melanocytes, which are cells that produce melanin (the pigment that gives skin its color). When melanocytes are less active, they produce less melanin, causing lighter skin (hypopigmentation). Sometimes, hypopigmentation is limited to smaller areas, like a birthmark or a scar. Certain infections, diseases, and conditions can cause hypopigmentation, too. Two conditions that have hypopigmentation as a symptom include:

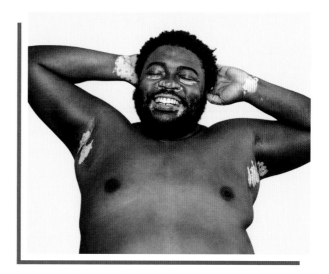

- ✦ **Vitiligo.** Millions of people have this autoimmune skin condition, where some melanocytes die or become completely inactive. When this happens, entire areas of the skin can turn white. Vitiligo is commonly found on the face and hands but can appear anywhere or spread all over, though it is not contagious. Vitiligo often begins to develop before the age of twenty. If you suspect you may have vitiligo, see your doctor. If you desire, there are treatments available that might help restore skin color.

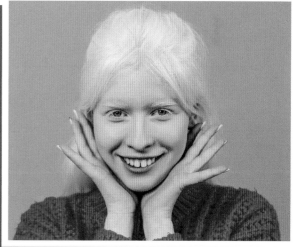

- ✦ **Albinism.** A genetic skin condition where the body produces no or very little melanin, which can result in hypopigmentation of the hair, eyes, and skin. The prefix *alb* means "white," referring to a person with albinism's lack of pigment.

Neither vitiligo nor albinism is contagious. See your doctor if you start noticing depigmentation on parts of your body, as there are some serious causes of hypopigmentation, such as certain types of skin cancer.

What Is Hyperpigmentation?

Hyperpigmentation is the opposite of hypopigmentation. When melanocytes are more active in certain areas, they produce more melanin, causing darker skin on those skin parts (hyperpigmentation).

No one can explain the precise cause of hyperpigmentation, which is when certain areas of skin are darker than others. Much of what determines the body's coloration is genetic. Some people, especially people of color, simply have more active melanocytes and are prone to hyperpigmentation spots, especially on the neck, in the armpits, and between the legs. Hyperpigmentation is also a sign used in screening for certain medical conditions, like diabetes or polycystic ovary syndrome (PCOS; see page 153).

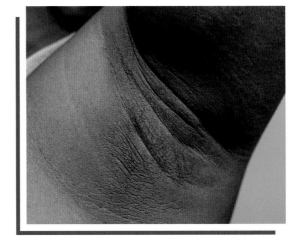

However, some specific situations can cause melanocytes to become hyperactive:

✦ **Sun exposure.** UV rays (from sunlight or a tanning bed) are a common cause of hyperpigmentation.

✦ **Friction and movement.** Tight shoes, chafing from places that naturally crease (like knees, elbows, and inner thighs), or too-tight underwear, jockstraps, or bra straps can cause skin darkening in these areas.

✦ **Skin damage.** Razor burn, popped pimples, scars, rashes, and other skin insults can cause hyperpigmentation.

It's normal for some body parts to appear darker than others, but there are a few things you can consider that might prevent hyperpigmentation:

- ✦ **Fit clothes and shoes properly.** Try wearing well-fitted shoes, bras, and underwear—not too tight! Friction from clothes can cause hyperpigmentation.

- ✦ **Limit skin damage.** Use proper hair-removal techniques (see page 61) and allow skin injuries to heal without picking at pimples or scabs.

- ✦ **Pamper yourself.** Exfoliate your skin in the shower (see page 15), and keep it moisturized, taking care to heavily lotion the darker spots, especially elbows and knees. Some people have luck covering up dark spots with body makeup or blending everything in with an all-over sunless tan.

Steer clear of creams marketed as "fading" or "bleaching." While they might lighten spots, they may contain harsh ingredients that can leave your skin dull and ashy, so avoid them unless under the supervision of a doctor.

If you notice parts of your skin darkening without friction or damage, see your doctor, as this can be a symptom of diabetes or another medical issue.

> Your nipples, anus, and genitalia all darken after puberty hormones surge. Some people think it's to make them more visible to possible romantic partners.

All about Rashes

A rash is when a section of skin becomes swollen or irritated. Rashes can develop when the skin gets extremely dry or because of a medical issue, like an allergy, infection, or noninfectious skin disease.

Rashes can appear anywhere on the body and are often discolored, itchy, and painful. In addition, they can come with raised bumps (like folliculitis), hives, and even blisters. Rashes can be temporary (anywhere from a few hours to a few months) or last for years—some become permanent.

If you find yourself faced with a rash that won't go away or appears frequently, don't try to diagnose yourself. Even though rashes can look very similar, they differ in origin. Fungal, bacterial, viral, and infestation rashes all can have a combination of itchy pimple-like bumps, welts, and scratches. Not only will the wrong medicines not work, but sometimes improper treatment makes your problems worse—for example, using an antibiotic meant for a bacterial infection might actually worsen a fungal infection. Nooooo!

When a rash pops up, keep a journal of everything you eat, drink, and put on your skin for a few weeks and how your skin reacts. This record can help to identify what works and doesn't work for your skin. Take this information to your doctor to help diagnose and treat your rash.

Rashes That Like to Stay

Three of the most common types of persistent, frequent skin rashes are eczema, psoriasis, and rosacea. These rashes can be hereditary, but they aren't contagious.

- ✦ **Eczema.** Also known as atopic dermatitis, eczema is a skin disorder often caused by a combination of internal inflammation, outside irritants and allergens, or other triggers. Eczema flare-ups can cause rashes anywhere from the scalp to the soles of feet—including genitalia. An eczema rash can be extremely itchy, causing sufferers to scratch even in their sleep, sometimes until the skin bleeds, which can lead to infection and more pain.

- ✦ **Psoriasis.** While external issues tend to contribute to flare-ups of eczema, psoriasis is an autoimmune disease caused when the body's immune system attacks itself. Like eczema, psoriasis rashes can be found anywhere on the body. However, they are usually only mildly uncomfortable.

- ✦ **Rosacea.** Rosacea is also an inflammatory skin disorder, meaning something external triggers it. Unlike eczema, rosacea is usually confined to the face, neck, and upper chest and tends to present with flushing of the skin, visible blood vessels, and acne-like bumps. Rosacea affects people differently. Some can't eat spicy foods; others can't be in the cold for too long. Even hormones can be a trigger, which is why many people find their cheeks burning nonstop during puberty. One trigger that seems to be universal is UV light, so be sure to always wear sunscreen of SPF 30 or higher daily.

Dozens of skin conditions can appear similar to eczema or psoriasis, and not everyone's skin reacts the same way to them or to possible remedies. See your doctor to get the right treatment for the right issue.

Rashes That Go Away

Other common but more short-term skin rashes include:

+ **Contact dermatitis.** Similar to atopic dermatitis (eczema), but only occurs at the exact point of contact with an irritant, triggering a physical reaction to a substance.

+ **Heat rash.** Triggered by . . . heat (surprise) and being outside in high temperatures.

+ **Drug rashes.** Triggered by prescribed oral (internally taken, like pills and liquids) and topical (ointments and lotions rubbed on the skin) medications.

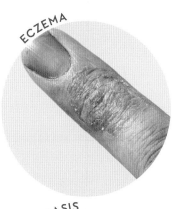

ECZEMA

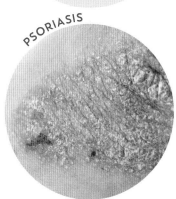

PSORIASIS

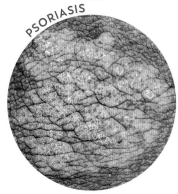

PSORIASIS

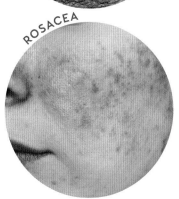

ROSACEA

+ **Chafing.** Wherever your skin touches other crevices or folds of skin, friction can cause a chafing rash in a variety of places: between your thighs, in your armpits, underneath your breasts, in your butt crack, and in rolls of fat on your stomach, back, or other parts of your body. Clothing, such as bras and bra straps, tight underwear, irritating seams, or small shoes, can also cause chafing on body parts like nipples, shoulders, genitalia, or feet. Moisture and warmth can worsen chafing and cause weeping wounds and odor. When chafing is more severe, it can become an inflammatory skin condition called intertrigo, which is commonly found in the armpit, under the breasts, and between the legs. Staying clean and dry can help prevent and heal chafing, so immediately after exercise or any other wet, sweaty activity, remove your clothes and shower. There are many over-the-counter lubricants, powders, and other products designed to help prevent and heal from chafing. Your doctor may also have some suggestions.

chafing

The Fungus Rash Is among Us!

No, a mushroom is not going to start sprouting from your back, but if you have a fungal infection, a common symptom is an annoying rash.

Two of the most common fungal infections are tinea and candida.

tinea

+ **Tinea.** It's called ringworm if it's on the neck, scalp, or face (even though it's a fungus and not a worm). If it's on the foot, it's called athlete's foot. If it's on or around the genitalia or thighs, it's called jock itch. While jock itch is more common on penises, it happens to people with vaginas, too. Tinea rashes tend to itch and can come with a potent smell—especially athlete's foot and jock itch. Sometimes tinea is paired with blisters that ooze white or yellow discharge.

+ **Candida.** Candida yeast infections are common on genitalia—in the vagina, on the scrotum, between thighs and stomach folds, underneath large breasts, on the penis head (known as balanitis), and even in the mouth and throat (called thrush). Symptoms include a rash that can itch and burn. White creamy and/or clumpy discharge with either no smell or a slightly yeasty (bread-like) odor may also appear.

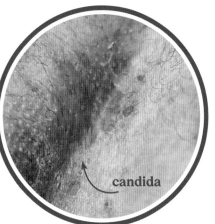

candida

Completely avoiding fungal infections isn't always possible, especially if you play sports (hence why common names for tinea are jock itch and athlete's foot). But anti-fungus tips are generally personal hygiene tips anyway, so remember to:

+ **Remove sweat (and sweaty stuff) ASAP.** Shower immediately after exercise (especially when you are physically touching other sweaty people) and change into clean clothes.

+ **Let your body breathe.** Go barefoot (or gloveless) to air out as much as possible. If you wear fake nails or nail polish, give your real nails a break for a few days after removing nails or polish before reapplying.

+ **Don't share personal items.** Fungal infections are often spread by sharing helmets, towels, loofahs, headbands, clothes, gloves, and shoes.

+ **Don't go barefoot in public places.** Flip-flops or other breathable shoes can keep foot fungus from being easily transmitted from the floors of pools, gyms, and locker rooms.

While over-the-counter treatments are available for fungal infections, it can be hard to get rid of them on your own. See your doctor, who can prescribe medication if necessary.

Nail Fungus

Some types of fungal infections, like nail infections (known as onychomycosis), can be caused by either tinea or candida. People with onychomycosis often have visible stains or spots on or underneath their fingernails or toenails that can be itchy, painful, and sometimes stinky. Nail fungus likes to breed in moist, dark environments like sweaty socks in shoes and acrylic fingernails that haven't been dried fully after

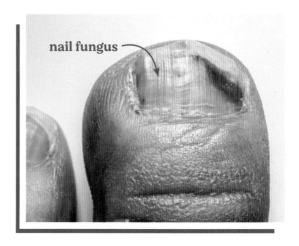

nail fungus

swimming or showering. Sharing gloves or shoes or stepping barefoot on the same shower floor as an infected person can also spread nail fungus. It's hard to get rid of nail fungus on your own, and clearing the infection completely can take a few months, so see your doctor to get the right medication for the type of infection you have. Your doctor can also screen for subungual melanoma, which is a skin cancer that looks a lot like nail fungus and is one of the most common skin cancers among people of color.

> Nails are made from the same proteins and structures as the skin.
> So is hair! A formal name for both nails and hair is "skin appendage."

Nail Fungus or Skin Cancer?

There's a sneaky cancer that looks a lot like nail fungus, called subungual melanoma. This specific type of cancer accounts for 75 percent of melanoma skin cancers found in African Americans—and is also the most common in Hispanic and Asian populations. Just another reason to get your nail fungus checked out as soon as you can!

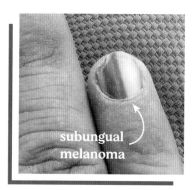
subungual melanoma

Ingrown Nails

Toenails or fingernails can improperly grow into the skin surrounding the nail and sometimes into the nail bed. This growth pattern is called an ingrown nail, and as it continues to grow, digging into your skin, it can become inflamed and very painful. Some causes of ingrown nails include:

+ **Improper cutting.** Nails should be cut straight across, not curved.

+ **Tight shoes.** Ingrown toenails are more common than fingernails due to poorly fitted shoes that push the nail toward the toe's skin.

+ **Genetics.** Ingrown nails can run in the family.

If you have an ingrown nail, don't ignore it. See your doctor. Especially if it looks infected! If you can't get to the doctor immediately, you can try a few things at home. If there's no infection, soak your hand or foot in warm water a few times a day for twenty minutes to help reduce swelling and make the nail bed softer. After soaking, keep the area around the ingrown nail clean and dry, and

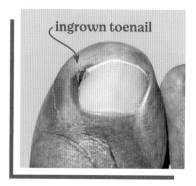
ingrown toenail

place a little cotton under the nail corner to keep it from growing inward (you can use the tip of an ear swab as well). Repeat this until the nail begins growing over the skin properly.

If the ingrown nail doesn't improve within a week, see your doctor because it may be something you can't fix on your own, and if it's allowed to continue growing in the wrong direction, serious and permanent damage can occur.

Are You a Nail-Biter?

You might bite your nails when nervous or removing a pesky hangnail, but if you are habitually doing so, it may be more than a nervous tic. Up to 30 percent of Americans are compulsive nail biters, unable to stop themselves from chewing even if it causes pain. In addition, extreme nail-biting, medically known as onychophagia, can be a sign of other issues, such as obsessive-compulsive disorder (OCD; see page 201 for more information). If you think you're suffering from severe nail-biting, see your doctor, who can examine you, prescribe medication, and/or refer you to a specialist if additional help is needed.

Calluses, Corns, and Bunions

Feet and hands often develop thickened areas of dead skin that form after an overload of friction or pressure, such as walking or running (especially barefoot) or frequent, repetitive movements like lifting weights, using tools, or playing an instrument. The most common types include:

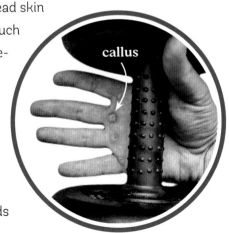
callus

+ **Calluses.** Painless patches that usually form on the soles of your feet and toes, the heels of your feet, and the palms of your hands or fingers. You can safely remove or improve the appearance of calluses by buffing them away with a pumice stone or using over-the-counter medicine. Scraping your feet with a razor at home is not wise, nor is getting your calluses scraped at a salon, as poor technique and/or dirty blades can lead to painful, dangerous infections and skin damage.

+ **Corns.** Painful, hardened bumps of skin (similar to a petrified blister) that frequently appear on the sides or tops of toes. They are generally smaller than calluses but are embedded deeper in the skin. This makes them difficult to remove or improve without a doctor's help.

corn

+ **Bunions.** Painful foot bumps that form when the long bone behind your big toe spreads and bends. Sometimes your bunion can develop calluses, too. Bunions are often passed down genetically or are a symptom of an injury or a disease, like diabetes, so see your doctor if you think you have one.

Anyone of any age can get a bunion, corn, or callus. They can sometimes be prevented on the feet by wearing socks with shoes that fit correctly. There are also corrective inserts for shoes. Gloves worn while using tools or performing manual labor can help to avoid or minimize hand calluses, as can the suggestions on page 39 on how to avoid hyperpigmentation. But some people just have hands and feet that are prone to them.

bunion

A podiatrist is a type of doctor who takes care of feet and foot injuries.

Problematic Skin Parasites

Sometimes, an itchy rash appears on your skin because of a parasite infestation. The word "infestation" sounds scary, but finding out that parasites have invited themselves to have a party on your skin is a pretty common occurrence. Millions of people become infested every single year . . . usually by each other!

Two common skin parasite infestations are scabies and lice, both of which can cause similar itchy, bumpy rashes that, when scratched, can become infected and even leave scars.

Scabies and lice are contagious—you get them from close contact with an already infested person or by sharing hats, pillows, hair tools, clothing, towels, or other personal items. So if someone you're sitting next to has lice, sometimes the bugs hop on over to you. Or, if you arm-wrestle someone infested with scabies, you might start scratching shortly thereafter. You can also spread either of these infestations during sexual activity.

Fortunately, although very annoying, neither scabies nor lice are life-threatening, though some lice can transmit illnesses and disease.

Scabies

Scabies mites are parasites that are invisible to the naked eye, but you can see and feel the annoying rash they leave behind as they burrow under your skin. Scabies can technically live anywhere on the body but tend to prefer burrowing between fingers and toes and other places where skin bends and folds. There's currently no over-the-counter medicine approved for scabies, so see your doctor for a prescription if you suspect an infestation.

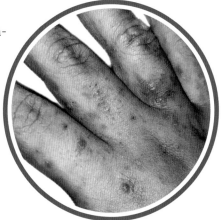

Lice

There are three types of lice, all of which are visible but very small parasites that feed off of human blood: body, head, and pubic lice.

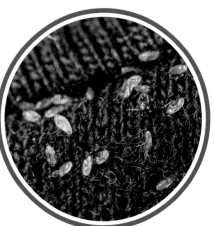

- **Body lice (seen in the magnified picture here).** The largest type of lice, body lice are about the size of a sesame seed. While head and pubic lice live on human bodies, body lice (despite their name) actually live in clothing and bedding.

- **Head lice.** These look similar to (and are just as itchy as) body lice but are smaller. They're usually seen moving around in the scalp. However, head lice and their eggs (called nits) can be found anywhere that hair grows, including occasionally in eyelashes and eyebrows.

- **Pubic lice.** These are the smallest species of lice. If you can see pubic lice, they look like teeny-tiny crabs (which is why "crabs" is a common nickname for them). While it's possible to catch pubic lice from unwashed infested bedding or other fabrics, it's usually caught during sexual activity.

How to Get Rid of Lice

A professional opinion is often needed to determine if an infestation rash is from scabies or lice, so if you can't figure it out from the following descriptions, see your doctor to make sure that you're treating the right parasite with the correct approach or medication.

Getting rid of lice tends to be time-consuming. First things first: prepare for a brief—but intense—lice war. It can often take a few hours to a couple of days working nonstop to kill enough lice and nits to avoid reinfestation.

Because adult lice can't survive more than one or two days away from a human body (the host), and lice eggs need the skin warmth to hatch, if you are careful and simultaneously clean your hair, bedding, clothing, and personal things very, very well, you'll likely end up exhausted but with the infestation extinguished.

Get lice off your skin and out of your hair. Since body lice live in clothing, a thorough shower should get rid of any stragglers on your skin. Getting lice out of your hair can be a bigger challenge, and there are three main ways to do so: over-the-counter products, manual removal of the lice and eggs, and prescription medicines.

+ **Over-the-counter products.** Lots of over-the-counter sprays, shampoos, and other treatments might kill lice. However, not all of them eliminate lice eggs, so they often can't completely solve your problem. There are also "super lice," which are resistant to traditional over-the-counter lice treatments.

+ **Manual removal of lice and eggs.** Combining an over-the-counter product with manual removal is a good first step. Combing through your hair with a specialized nitpicking comb designed to remove lice and, most importantly, sticky lice eggs is very effective when done correctly. There are professionals you can pay to comb your hair for you if you prefer. This tedious combing is best done on very wet and well-conditioned hair to avoid damage and discomfort.

+ **Prescription medicines.** Your doctor might be able to prescribe stronger medicines that work better on super lice and that also kill eggs.

Get lice out of your stuff. After you've cleared your head, sanitize anything you might have touched while infested. Gather all washable clothes and bed linens you've used recently and wash them in hot water. Items you've had contact with that can't be washed should either be placed in the clothes dryer on high heat for twenty minutes or bagged up for a week or two to starve the lice and any eggs that hatch.

STEP 3

Repeat a few days later. A few days after the first round of hair- and stuff-cleaning, it is wise to follow up with a second round, just to be sure you got everything before additional eggs hatch. Lice infestations are easier to eradicate when there are just a few lice, but once they start multiplying, it's harder to stop.

Note that if you are sexually active and find scabies, lice, or lice nits in your nethers, it's important to see your doctor as you likely need to be tested for other STIs.

head hair & body hair

Did you know that porcupine quills are a type of hair? Dog whiskers and fur are hair, too. All mammals have some hair somewhere, and while people evolved to lose most hair a long time ago, a lot remains on our heads and bodies. And thank goodness!

When you think about your own hair, you're probably focused on how to style or remove it. But hair exists for more than just appearance.

The hair on your scalp, face, and body has a variety of functions, including:

✦ Defending our bodies from injury, infection, and cancer-causing UV rays. For example, without eyebrows, sweat and rain would travel straight down your forehead into your eyes, making it difficult to see.

✦ Regulating our body temperature

✦ Helping us touch and feel. Some hairs are even more responsive to touch than our skin.

All over your body, up to five million follicles sprout up to four strands of hair each. The only places on your body that never grow hair are your nails, belly button, lips, the palms of your hands, and the bottoms of your feet. Because your body can't re-place hair follicles lost from injury, scarred skin cannot grow hair.

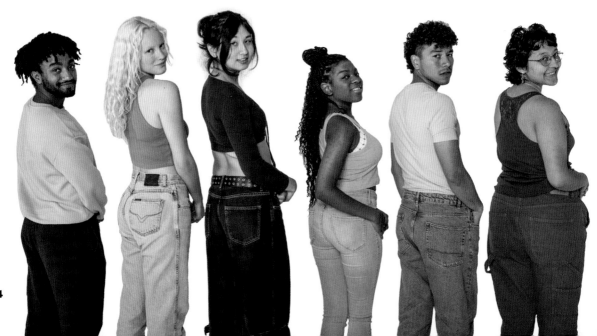

Is Hair Actually Dead?

By the time you can see strands of hair, it's already dead. That's why it doesn't hurt to cut hair!

Before hair erupts through the skin, each strand goes through a growing phase. After growth stops, the hair dies and rests in the follicle for a few months before eventually falling out to make room for new hair to grow in the same follicle.

The more time hair stays in the growing phase, the longer it can become. All hair grows at a rate of about half an inch each month. Genetics and ethnicity can play a part in whether it grows faster or slower, as can weather—hair grows faster in warmer months. Stress can affect hair growth, too. Because of haircuts, hair removal, and hair damage (like split ends), sometimes you don't see evidence of new length, but your hair's growth cycle is always continuing.

While all hair grows at about the same rate each month, the amount of time each strand grows before dying is different for each body part. This resting growth phase (telogen phase) can take a few weeks to a few years. Head hair has the longest growing phase—it can continue to grow for up to six years. Beard hair can also grow for years. The rest of your body hair only gets a few weeks or months of growing time—that's why your body hair, like eyelashes and eyebrows, are so short.

> Ever wonder how older people can often grow such long, white beards? Scientists have found evidence that white beard hair can grow up to four times faster than beard hair that hasn't gone gray yet!

Vellus or Terminal?

There are two types of hair: vellus and terminal.

Vellus hair is the nearly invisible fine fuzz, or "peach fuzz," that lightly covers most of your body. When puberty starts, testosterone and other hormones transform some vellus hair into terminal hair. (See page 164 for more on hormones.)

Terminal hair is the thicker, darker, denser, and longer body hair found on the armpits, legs, and crotch of most postpuberty people.

Your scalp hair, eyelashes, and eyebrows are terminal hairs, too.

Terminal Hair Can Be Everywhere!

People born with penises usually produce more masculinizing hormones like testosterone, so more of their vellus hair can turn into terminal hair all over the body, including on the face, back, upper thighs, stomach, chest . . . even on the tops of feet.

It's also (but not always) possible to grow full mustaches and beards. It's totally normal for facial hair to grow in patches—so if you are looking forward to growing a beard, know that it can take years for all your facial hair to "connect," and sometimes it never does. Keeping facial hair well moisturized and using grooming tools—like small scissors for trimming, a beard brush, and waxes and balms made especially for facial hair—can help with appearance while you wait for additional growth. Some people find that colored fillers, like pencils and powders, can help hide specific spots.

Uh, I Was Not Expecting to Grow a Mustache!

People born with vaginas usually produce less testosterone and other hormones that ramp up terminal hair transformation, so terminal hair tends to cover less than a third of their bodies. That said, with so much hair all over the body, there are bound to be some patches that pop up in surprising places.

Many people find that darker, thicker hair can develop not just in the crotch area, armpits, and legs but also on the chin and upper lip. When terminal hair unexpectedly shows up as more than a few stray hairs on the face, chest, stomach, hands, and feet, there might be a hormone imbalance, like polycystic ovary syndrome (PCOS; see page 153 for more). If you're developing more body or facial hair than you expect, see your doctor, They can run blood tests and visually inspect your body and facial hair to determine whether it's truly excessive (and might be a condition called hirsutism).

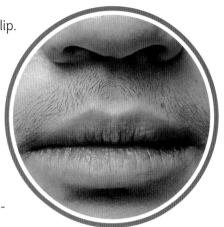

Certain medicines, including gender-affirming hormone therapy, can affect your terminal hair growth. People who take masculinizing hormones may find their facial and body hair thickening, and people who take feminizing hormones often report their body and facial hair become less noticeable. More on sex and gender starts on page 163.

Scalp Hair Changes, Too!

As puberty hormones transform your body, they can change your scalp hair, too. Some people are born blond but turn brunette by high school. Others have straight hair as toddlers but supertight coils after puberty. Even if hair changes aren't that intense, many people see some difference in the color, thickness, and texture of head hair at various stages of life. Pregnancy and illnesses can change your scalp hair . . . for example, many cancer survivors find their hair looks very different than before chemotherapy.

Normally, around 100,000 strands of hair sprout from the follicles in your scalp.

Shoulder Snow

Is it snowing on your shoulders? The word "dandruff" actually means "itch-dirt," and it describes the buildup—and flaking off—of skin cells on your scalp.

Dandruff can feel dry or wet. Dry dandruff is usually white or translucent and feels powdery or scaly. When the scalp's dead skin cells mix with scalp oils, dandruff becomes "wet" and yellow, forming larger, more noticeable clumps. Dandruff can also cause your scalp to smell.

Dandruff can happen for various reasons, many of which are contradictory. It's stressful trying to determine the cause, and that stress can also increase the amount of dandruff you produce! A dry scalp can cause dandruff, as can having an oily scalp. Washing your hair too much or not enough can also cause it. UV rays from sunlight might help limit dandruff, but sun exposure can also cause dandruff. Finally, it can be seasonal and more common in the winter.

dandruff

Sometimes, your scalp shedding isn't dandruff but dried leftover hair products. Because everyone's dandruff is different, look at your personal habits and see what might need to change.

- ✦ Are you washing your hair too much or not enough?

- ✦ Can you lower your levels of stress?

- ✦ Do you need to wear a hat to protect your hair from the sun or cold air?

- ✦ Are you using too many products or the wrong type of products for your particular scalp and hair?

Scientists believe that a scalp fungus could be behind some types of dandruff, so an antifungal treatment might help. Coconut oil is a natural antifungal that may improve dandruff if you rub a dime-sized amount into your scalp every day. Look for 100 percent coconut oil and not just hair products that are coconut-scented.

Over-the-counter shampoos specifically for dandruff often include antifungal medicines and antifungal essential oils, like tea tree oil. There are dozens of anti-dandruff shampoos, conditioners, and hair creams, many of which use ingredients that can react differently or reveal side effects depending upon your specific scalp. For example, one product a friend loves may worsen your dandruff, but another that no one else gets results from might completely control it.

See a dermatologist if you're still finding flakes after trying different remedies. A doctor can examine your scalp and prescribe a stronger shampoo or suggest additional treatments. They can also see if you have a more severe problem like psoriasis (see page 40), ringworm (page 42), or seborrheic dermatitis, which is when dandruff comes with scalp irritation and inflammation. Seborrheic dermatitis can also be found in other hairy areas, like your eyebrows, upper lip, and even chest hair.

Dandruff, psoriasis, and seborrheic dermatitis are not contagious, though each can be embarrassing to deal with. But don't feel bad! Up to half of all people will suffer the fate of itchy, flaky dandruff at some point in their lives, so you're absolutely not alone.

Hair Loss Happens

It's normal to shed about a hundred and fifty hairs each day, but sometimes our hair falls out more than usual. Reasons include:

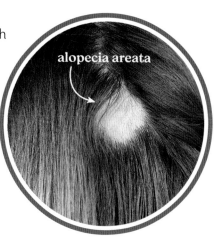

alopecia areata

+ Stress

+ Illness and certain medications

+ Nutritional deficiencies from extreme dieting

+ Damage from hairstyles, hair products, or hair chemicals

- ✦ Autoimmune diseases like alopecia areata (as seen in the picture in this section), which tend to appear before a person turns thirty and cause bald spots to pop up on your body and scalp

- ✦ Genetics and hormone fluctuations. Some people, especially people born with penises and people who take masculinizing gender-affirming hormones, have a type of alopecia called androgenetic alopecia, where some hair follicles shrink over time in a certain pattern, causing hair thinning and eventually baldness. People who have recently given birth also sometimes experience temporary hair thinning and loss due to hormones.

Sometimes hair loss stops, either once the cause has been established or just on its own, even if it's an autoimmune disease. However, figuring out the cause of your hair loss can help you slow it down or prevent it from happening in the future, and the earlier, the better. A dermatologist can help you diagnose what's going on and recommend treatment options.

Healthy Hair Habits

Because every scalp has different sensitivities, there's no one way to maintain a healthy head of hair. That said, there are a few steps you can take to help take good care of your head hair.

- ✦ **Check your sleeping style.** Hair breakage can be caused by sleeping with tangled or wet hair, or even by the fabric of your pillowcase. Consider investing in a silk or satin pillowcase or a hair bonnet for protection, especially if your hair is curly or coily.

- ✦ **Check your routines.** Are you over-styling your hair with heat or color? How often do you wash your hair? Maybe you wash it too much for your hair type, or not enough. Do you brush too hard, which can cause oil overproduction, or not enough, which leaves your strands knotty and dry?

+ **Check your ends.** While it can seem contradictory, cutting your hair a little bit every couple of months can help it grow. The ends of your hair are prone to splitting, especially if you have dry or low-porosity hair. Split ends usually travel up the hair shaft, so they'll do a lot more damage to your hair's overall length and look if you don't trim them in time.

+ **Check your products.** Everyone's hair reacts differently to certain ingredients— what makes someone else's hair perfectly shiny may make yours flaky, frizzy, dull, or greasy.

+ **Check the weather.** Cold weather tends to make hair drier, and hot and humid weather can cause hair to become oilier (though for some people, it can be the reverse). Wearing a hat to protect your hair from the elements can help avoid dryness and damage from cold winds and hot rays.

Hair Removal

There's no one type of hair styling or removal that is "good" or "bad." What you choose to do with the hair on your head and body can be a practical decision, a personal statement, or nothing at all—you decide.

If you do want to rid yourself of facial or body hair, there are a variety of techniques you can use, including:

+ **Shaving.** One or more sharp blades cut hair as close to the skin as possible. It is one of the easiest, fastest, and least expensive ways to remove hair and can be used successfully on any body part. Hair tends to grow back in a few days, though you can sometimes feel regrowth (called stubble) as soon as a few minutes after shaving. To avoid razor burn—when the razor blade nicks skin, causing a painful rash—try to shave only in the shower or right after, as warm water opens pores, softens skin, and helps razors glide smoothly. It's important to always use a sharp, fresh blade. If you're using an electric shaver, make sure it's clean.

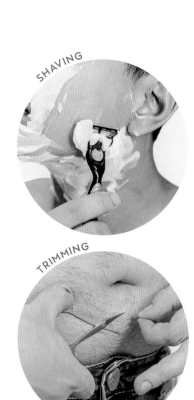

Face shaving with a razor can be tricky—every angle around your nose, jaw, and chin is a new opportunity to nick yourself, which can cause bleeding (and pain). To nix shaving nicks, try using shaving cream or gel, which helps razor blades glide smoothly over the skin. Shaving a wet face can also help minimize friction, thus leading to fewer cuts. If you do all this and still end up wounded, apply pressure to the nick with a clean, wet cloth for thirty to forty-five seconds. This helps the blood clot so you can get on with your day without a piece of toilet paper or a bandage adhered to your face.

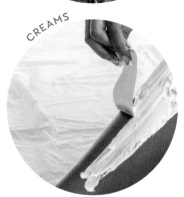

+ **Trimming.** Using small scissors to snip hairs (ideally ones made specifically for hair trimming, like the pair in this picture) can be a good option, especially for people with skin that is sensitive or when full removal isn't desired. Trimming eliminates the risk of razor

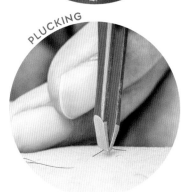

burn and ingrown hairs (razor bumps). You can trim hair anywhere, but it's particularly useful for nose and pubic hair. Sometimes trimming longer hair before using other hair-removal methods like waxing or shaving can make the process easier.

✦ **Creams, lotions, and powders.** Hair-removal potions are chemical compounds that dissolve hair at the surface. Often called depilatories (though that term refers to all forms of hair removal generally), chemical removal is a painless way to eliminate unwanted hair. People prone to razor burn and ingrown hairs often find that their skin feels smoother when using depilatories. Depilatories can be used anywhere there's hair—including beards and mustaches, and the results last as long as shaving. The downside is they can be smelly and messy. Plus, depilatories can easily cause rashes and burns, so take extra care if you have sensitive skin, and never leave the product on too long. Before using, you should test a small patch on a hidden body part to see how your skin reacts.

✦ **Plucking and epilation.** The manual removal of individual hairs from the follicle is called plucking or tweezing. Because this technique pulls out the entire hair, root and all, the area usually stays hair-free longer than shaving. It can be time-consuming to remove every individual hair, so tweezing is best left to stray hairs or sparsely covered areas, like your chin, toes, or eyebrows. Mechanical or electric tweezers that grip multiple hairs at once are called epilators, and their efficiency makes it possible to pluck areas with more hair, like legs and underarms. Make sure to pluck or epilate hair in the direction it grows, and try not to dig into the skin, as improper tweezing can cause scarring, pitting, and ingrown hairs.

✦ **Threading.** Using two pieces of thin string to remove entire rows of hair at a time is a speedier version of tweezing that's less expensive than waxing. Threading salons have popped up all across America and are popular for facial hair removal, especially on eyebrows. Like with waxing and tweezing, threaded body parts stay smoother for longer than if you shave. Make sure your threader uses new thread and that your skin is cleaned to avoid infection, as sometimes threading can nick the skin, causing it to bleed—keep an eye out for any other complications that may arise. Because irritation from the constant string tugging can cause puffiness and reddening of the skin, prepare a cool compress to use on your skin directly after to reduce inflammation. People with sensitive skin should try a small area of hair, like the chin, before going for full-face threading.

THREADING

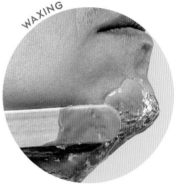

WAXING

+ **Waxing.** Manual removal of a large number of hairs from root to tip using a sticky substance is possible with waxing. Beeswax is one common ingredient, but other substances like rosin, sugar, and honey can be used, too. "Soft" wax requires cloth or paper strips to adhere to the wax on your skin before being ripped off, while "hard" wax dries when cooled and can be pulled off your skin directly. Uniquely, waxing removes not only the hair in the area but also the top layer of dead skin cells, giving the skin a very soft look and feel. It's hard, but not impossible, to wax yourself, though complications like burns from the wax being too hot can occur. Also, it's a learned skill to be able to self-inflict the pain that comes with ripping off the hair—and one you might never be able to master!

Some people may opt to use a cream to bleach their body hair instead of removing it. While bleaching doesn't remove hair, it makes it nearly invisible on lighter skin tones. Even though bleaching is permanent, the hair continues to grow, so it must be redone every few weeks. In addition, some people are allergic to bleaching chemicals, so a patch test is necessary before slathering your entire body with bleaching cream. And even if you want your carpet to match your drapes, avoid DIY bleaching in your pubic area, as having harsh chemicals down there can cause skin irritation or even burns.

+ **Semi-permanent medical hair removal.** If you really can't stand DIY hair removal and have money to burn (hair off), medical hair-removal techniques like electrolysis, light therapy, and laser treatments can kill individual hairs at the root. While there are at-home medical hair-removal devices, it's safest to have these services done by licensed professionals like dermatologists and estheticians. That way, you avoid burns and scarring. Make sure to check the professional's references before you go, and pay attention to their technique as they work on your body. Often, this removal is permanent, but sometimes the hair does return (especially if you haven't finished going through puberty or are having hormonal shifts, like in pregnancy), and there are no refunds on these expensive procedures. People with darker skin tones should be especially careful when choosing permanent hair removal, as darker skin is more prone to scarring, pigmentation changes, or technique failure.

Ingrown Hairs

Hair that is temporarily removed eventually starts to regrow. As the individual hairs erupt through the skin, some might retreat back into their follicles, especially in areas that grow curlier, thicker hair. This can cause bumps called ingrown hairs, also known as razor bumps.

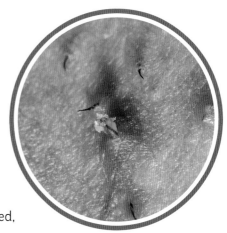

When ingrown hairs become infected or inflamed,

it's a type of folliculitis. Ingrown hairs or folliculitis can happen anywhere there's hair, from your face to your toes, but are especially common in moist crevices like armpits and around your genitals.

Like pimples from acne, you do NOT want to pop ingrown hairs, even though it's tempting. Scarring from poorly handled ingrown hairs and folliculitis is very common. Less is more when it comes to healing bumpy skin—stopping all hair removal for a few weeks, leaving the skin alone, and waiting for the bumps to go away on their own is often the best plan of action. If the ingrown hair doesn't improve and instead becomes more painful, swollen, or oozy, see your doctor, as you may have an infection.

You can take steps to prevent ingrown hairs in the future. Gentle exfoliation helps remove dead cells on the outer layer of your skin that might cause hair to curl back into the follicle. Right before hair removal and for a few days after, use a washcloth or loofah to gently scrub the area. An exfoliating product can be fun to use, too—see page 15 for an exfoliation recipe.

> People today often prefer to purposefully remove their pubic hair, but back in the seventeenth century, a heap of pubic hair was a sign of great health. Lice infestations and complications from sexually transmitted infections (STIs) caused many people to have to remove the hair on their genitals. So, to veil any signs of venereal diseases, special custom-made pubic wigs called merkins became popular.

Hair-Pulling Disorder

Many of us reach for a pair of tweezers and pluck a stray hair or two that's bothering us, but sometimes, hair pulling becomes compulsive. This is called trichotillomania or hair-pulling disorder. Trichotillomania usually starts between ten and thirteen years of age, though it can be triggered at any time. It's estimated to affect up to 1 out of every 50 people, and people with trichotillomania often also have dermatillomania, or skin-picking disorder (see page 23 for more).

Even though hair pulling is a physical act, it's a mental health issue that fits within the obsessive-compulsive spectrum. As it's difficult to solve a mental health issue on your own, seek professional help (see page 198 for types of therapists). The faster that treatment starts for hair pulling, the better the chances you'll be able to develop coping mechanisms and strategies to stop.

chests
&
breasts

Everyone knows humans are mammals, but did you know the word "mammals" comes from the Latin word for breast, *mamma*? That's because one of the defining elements of mammals is our ability to grow milk-producing breasts. And of the five thousand mammals on Earth, humans are the only ones that develop permanent breasts well before they are needed to feed babies.

All people, regardless of genitalia, are born with flat chests that contain undeveloped mammary glands. If developed (matured), tiny tube-like milk ducts in these glands can carry the breast milk out of the body through the nipple.

Everyone's chests start to mature when puberty jump-starts the production of hormones like estrogen and testosterone (see page 164 for more on hormones).

As discussed on page 165, people born with vaginas usually produce a lot more estrogen than testosterone, so there's not much of an increase in muscle mass in the chest area. Instead, there's more glandular tissue development and a significant increase in breast fat. Estrogen also matures the mammary glands and milk ducts, making it possible to produce breast milk.

People born with penises usually produce a lot more testosterone than estrogen, so puberty tends to cause very little permanent chest fat development (though a little—or a lot—of temporary chest fat is very common during puberty; see page 79 for more on growing unexpected breasts). Instead, testosterone significantly increases muscle mass, filling out pectoral muscles and widening the shoulders and chest.

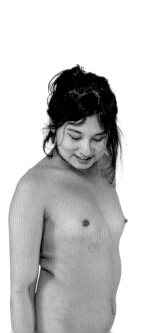
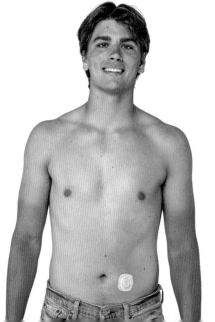
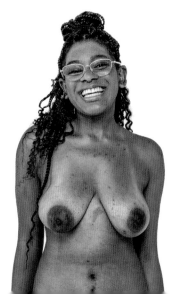

> Chests and breasts also function as erogenous zones, meaning they feel really good when touched.

Self-Consciousness about Chests and Breasts

Chests and breasts come in all shapes and sizes and do not define your worth. Yet it's very easy to get emotionally caught up in what your chest looks like. Many, many people feel unhappy about the size of their chest, whether it's the muscles they're concerned about, the breasts, or both. Too big? Too small? It's almost never just right!

Since these changes are front and center (literally), it can feel like your chest is getting a lot of attention, which might make you self-conscious, especially if people start to treat you differently because of something you can't control (see page 167 for more on this frustrating aspect of growing up).

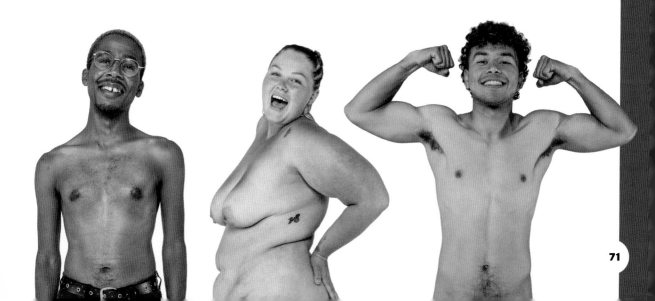

Plus, it can be hard enough dealing with expected chest changes, like nipple darkening and stretch marks, but it's especially difficult to remain calm when unexpected changes happen during puberty. Common surprises include leaky nipples (see page 75) or unexpected breasts (page 79), which sprout up on more than half of people born with penises.

Fortunately, this manual is here to help you de-stress about your changing chest!

Is Areola Another Name for Nipple?

Nope! What you probably call "nipples" actually have two parts: the areola *and* the nipple. Your areolas are the round-ish areas around your nipples, and most people are born with two of each. Very rarely, someone is born with congenital athelia, a condition where one or both nipples and areolas are missing.

third nipple

Some of us are born with one or more "accessory" nipples, medically known as polythelia and commonly referred to as having a third (or fourth, or fifth) nipple. Sometimes, areolas also grow alongside the extra nipple(s), and occasionally a full breast grows around the extra nipple—this is called polymastia. Tell your doctor if you have an extra nipple or breast so they can monitor it, as sometimes extra nipples are also associated with other health concerns, like kidney disease and cancer.

Areolas

Areolas usually are a different, darker color than the rest of your body's skin, but not always. They can range in size from as small as a dime to as big as a teacup. Every size and shape (including puffy) is normal! During puberty, even though estrogen is

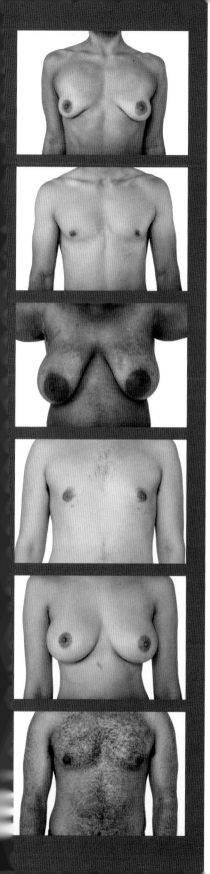

the main hormone that triggers breast development, even people born with penises and testicles can grow larger, puffy nipples that tend to go away after a few years, though sometimes they do not (see page 79 for more on gynecomastia).

The texture of areolas tends to differ from the surrounding skin. Most areolas are covered in little bumps called Montgomery's glands. Some people have a few Montgomery's glands, while others have a lot. These glands produce and release a tiny amount of antibacterial oil that protects and cleans the nipple.

When they're healthy, Montgomery's glands are totally painless. If they get blocked with oil or dead skin cells, they can become sore, red, and swollen. But though they might look like a pimple, they're not! Don't try to pop them or use acne medication, as this could cause irritation, scarring, or an infection. Eventually, they will probably go back to normal if you simply leave the areola alone and keep it clean and dry. If it sticks around for more than a week, or if your Montgomery's glands frequently become hard, swollen, or painful, see your doctor.

> Sometimes hair grows on the areola.
> The section on body hair starts on p. 53.

Nipples

In the center of your areolas are your nipples. Nipples also come in all colors, shapes, and sizes. Some look like pencil erasers, others are the size of bottle caps, and some nipples are barely there. When breastfeeding, the tip of the nipple is where most breast milk is expressed.

Most people's nipples protrude, meaning they stick out slightly from the surrounding areola. When one or both protruding areolas are stimulated—by cold, touch, excitement, or even a gentle breeze—tiny muscles inside your chest contract, which can cause the areola to shrink and nipples to harden and protrude even more. When stimulation stops, most nipples return to their normal state.

Some people's nipples always protrude, whether stimulated or not, and that's normal, too.

Preventing Nipple Chafe

Protruding nipples are prone to chafing, like rubbing up against clothing, making the nipple sore. Chest sweat can make chafing worse, as can movement from athletic activities.

When a nipple chafes for too long, there can be discharge or even blood. For example, marathon runners can suffer from "runner's nipple," where their nipples are so irritated after rubbing against clothing for hours that they bleed uncontrollably.

Layering tops, wearing well-fitting bras with cups made of thicker material, and even carefully applying adhesive bandages or nipple concealers (found at most drugstores) can help neutralize nipple chafing. Make sure to cover your nipple with the nonadhesive part, and when it's time to remove, pull slowly; then moisturize the skin after to help it recover. Never use duct tape or products with other strong adhesives

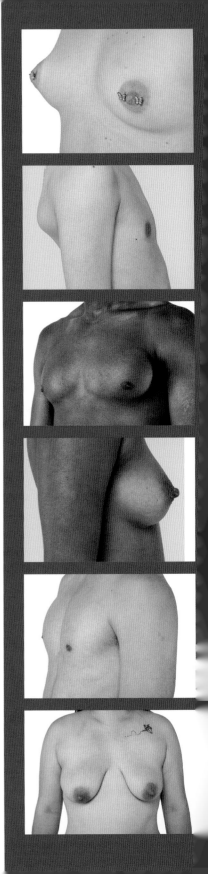

near your nipple. To soothe chafed nipples, carefully rub in an emollient like petroleum jelly to help the skin heal. It can also help to rub in an emollient before placing bandages over the nipple.

Hey! Where's My Nipple?

Some people's nipples never "stick out," or protrude. Up to 1 in every 5 people are born with at least one flat or inverted nipple, meaning that the nipple never "pops out" but stays flat or points inward, no matter the temperature or stimulation.

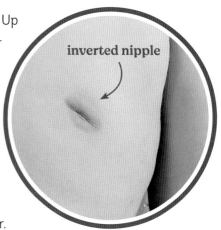
inverted nipple

There are no medical issues related to people who are born with inverted nipples, and an inverted nipple often starts protruding during puberty. However, if you find that one or both of your usually pointy nipples spontaneously inverts, see your doctor.

Nip Drips

If you see something drip from your nip, don't panic, even if you're a person born with a penis. When any liquid leaks from a nipple (and you're not breastfeeding) it can be alarming, but it's rather common—up to 25 percent of people may experience galactorrhea, which is nipple discharge that has nothing to do with breastfeeding. Puberty can cause leaky nipples on anyone, thanks to the surge of hormones happening that the body hasn't figured out how to sort yet. (Nipple discharge is also common for people who unexpectedly grow breasts; see page 79 for more.)

Infections and certain medications, like some prescription drugs and hormonal birth control, can cause nipple discharge. Nipple chafing from clothing can also cause discharge. Very rarely, nipple discharge can be a sign of breast cancer in any person, especially if it is bloody. See page 86 for more on breast cancer prevention.

If "nip drip" happens to you, do not squeeze. Keep the nipple clean and dry, stop using lotions or perfume near the breast area, and see your doctor immediately.

Growing Chest Pains

It's normal for all people going through puberty to have chests and breasts that sometimes feel sore or itchy, whether all over or just around the nipple. Often, it's just growing pains—either from working out or breast development. Sometimes chafing (see page 42) or allergic reactions to the clothing you wear over your nipples (top, undershirt, binder, or bra), or the soap used to clean your clothes, might be causing discomfort. Or, if you recently shaved your chest, you could be dealing with ingrown hairs or razor burn (pages 65 and 62).

Over-the-counter pain medication and alternating hot and cold compresses can help with pain and inflammation. If chest pain doesn't go away or is accompanied by difficulty breathing, a lump, nipple discharge, or heat radiating from the area, or if you're concerned that something else might be causing the pain, see your doctor.

The Quest for Muscular Chests

Since testosterone is the main hormone that triggers chest muscle development, the chests of people born with penises tend to become more muscular when puberty begins (see page 164 for more). The main chest muscles, called your pectoralis muscles, or "pecs" for short, are beneath the skin of your nipples and areolas. Pecs are the largest muscles in the chest.

Chest shape is determined by not just muscles but also bone structure and where body fat is stored. Some people are born with a chest that tends to develop more fat than others, resulting in a softer, rounder chest and abdomen, both pre- and postpuberty. Your family's genetics can also determine how easy it is for you to increase the size of your chest muscles—some people have body types with pecs that easily puff up with strength training, while others do not.

Chests naturally vary in appearance, just like breasts. But even when we know no one type of body is better than another, social media (and society at large) can encourage unrealistic, difficult-to-attain-and-maintain ideas of what a "manly" chest should look like. For people who want to appear masculine and strong, the pressure to build a big, muscular chest can feel very intense.

For some, the struggle to be very muscular and big-chested can become all-consuming, leading to a body dysmorphic disorder called muscle dysphoria, also known as bigorexia. Similar to how a person with anorexia thinks their body is too big, people with bigorexia feel their body is not big enough. Bigorexia sufferers spend excessive time worrying about and working on beefing up their bodies, and there's often a disconnect between the person's actual body and what their mind tells them about their body. For example, a recent study found that many bodybuilders considered themselves smaller and weaker than others, even though it was factually untrue.

The teen years are often when the first signs of bigorexia show up. Here are some questions you can ask yourself if you suspect you might be suffering from bigorexia:

+ Do you think your chest is too small?

+ Do you think your body is too thin and wish you could be heavier?

+ Do you wish you were stronger?

+ Do you wear loose-fitting clothes so that no one can see your body?

+ Do you hate your body?

+ Do you think your legs are too thin?

+ Do you work out excessively?

+ Do you feel anxious or depressed when you miss a day of exercise?

+ Are you embarrassed to let people see you without a shirt?

✦ Do you cancel social activities or miss opportunities because of your workout schedule?

If you have some of these thoughts some of the time, that's perfectly normal—everyone does. It's when these thoughts take over your life, weighing on you daily, making you feel bad about yourself, and completely chipping away at your confidence, that they might be considered symptoms of bigorexia.

Bigorexia sufferers may look healthy on the outside but often suffer high levels of anxiety, depression, substance abuse, and suicidal thoughts and behaviors. If you answered "yes" to many of the questions in the previous list, talk to a trusted adult or see your doctor, who can fully assess you. Talk therapy can also help you work through your feelings.

> Stretch marks on your chest and breasts are common. Because growth often happens in this area rather rapidly, the skin doesn't have time to stretch properly, resulting in small tears in the skin's middle layer. While stretch marks rarely disappear completely, they do fade over time. See page 32 for more on stretch marks, medically referred to as striae gravidarum.

Sunken Chests

Pectus excavatum, also known as sunken chest syndrome, is a very common chest condition. People born with penises are five times more likely to have a sunken chest, but anyone can be born with the syndrome. For most people, it is just a way in which they look different from others. However, some people might have trouble with self-esteem or other problems with their health, depending upon the severity of the condition. If you

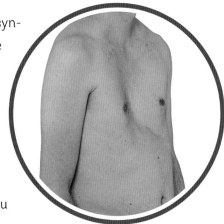

see yourself in this example chest, know that you are not alone. Physical complications from pectus excavatum, like fatigue and chest pain, can become more of an issue over time (especially in the tween and teen years), so see your doctor, who can check out your chest and offer support.

I Was Not Expecting Breasts!

You might be surprised to learn that half of people born with penises will develop some visible breast tissue on one or both sides of their chest by the time they are fourteen years old (like the fifteen-year-old person in this photo). This is often due

to a medical condition called gynecomastia—and is related to the body producing more-than-expected amounts of estrogen. The resulting hormone imbalance can cause breast tissue growth on either or both sides of the chest. Nipples and areolas can enlarge and become puffy as well.

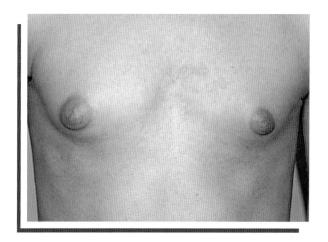

Gynecomastia can happen at any life stage, but puberty is the most common time. Usually breast tissue that develops during puberty goes away in a few months to a few years, whenever the body's hormones settle down. Occasionally, it can take longer, and sometimes it is permanent.

Some medical conditions and medicines can also stimulate breast growth, and people with intersex variations assigned male at birth may develop breast tissue during puberty. (See page 165 for more on intersex variations and page 164 for more on sex assigned at birth.) You cannot self-diagnose gynecomastia or other medical conditions, and people get gynecomastia all the time, but if it happens to you, you might feel like you're the only one with this condition or that something's wrong with you.

But the stats show that you're probably in the majority! See your doctor, who can screen for different issues and discuss treatment options, if desired. Don't let shame keep you from getting answers to any questions and concerns you might have. Also, talking to a therapist can help manage the emotions and feelings that might come with having this condition (see page 189 for types of therapists).

Pendulous Breasts

Many people think that perky, round, and gravity-defying breasts are the only kind of breasts that puberty brings on, but that's not true. Often when breasts start to develop, they pop out in a different shape than expected. Surprise! A lot of people born with vaginas grow breasts that hang with a natural sag or droop when braless, especially larger and heavier ones. When breasts carry more weight near the areola and nipple, gravity pulls the breasts downward, which can cause them to droop and even swing. Sometimes the areola and nipple point downward. Pendulous breasts are completely normal and very common, even among teenagers. While exercise can enhance the body's overall tone (and it's great anyway for self-care), there's not a specific breast-lift exercise that 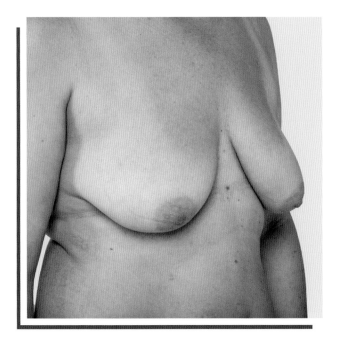 can make much of a difference with pendulous breasts. But before considering surgery for this perfectly normal and healthy breast shape, check out the magic of a properly fitted and supportive bra, many of which can create the illusion of breast perkiness no magician could match. (See page 89 for more on bras.)

Barely There Breasts

Sometimes, a person born with a vagina might see areola and nipple darkening and growth without much breast enlargement, even if other expected signs of maturity, such as pubic hair and menstrua-tion, have shown up. It's a perfectly normal, healthy, and common body type to have smaller breasts all throughout adulthood. However, breast growth can happen well into a person's twenties or even later, depending upon a variety of fac-tors, including weight gain, certain medicines, and pregnancy. So don't be surprised if you suddenly start to sprout bigger breasts!

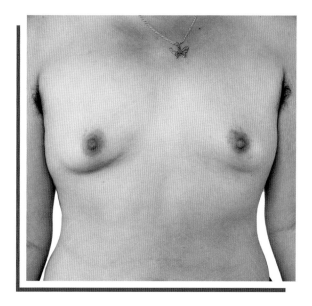

Sometimes very athletic peo-ple, frequent dieters, or people with poor eating habits may not get enough of the nutrients and calories needed to grow breasts. In these cases, breast development may restart when athletic activity slows down or nutrition im-proves.

Several medical conditions can affect breast growth; for example, some people with intersex variations assigned female at birth may develop very small or no breasts during puberty. (See page 164 for more on sex assigned at birth and page 165 for more on intersex variations.) If you aren't developing breast tissue that you were ex-pecting, see your doctor, who can examine you and discuss available tests that can help figure out what's going on.

People who want larger breasts should note that no matter what anyone says, sleep positions, breast massages, and specific foods or drinks will not make a signifi-cant difference in breast growth.

One Breast Is Bigger Than the Other

Anything that you have more than one of on your body is *rarely* going to be exactly the same size, even if the difference is barely noticeable. One of your ears is a bit bigger, one of your feet is a tad tinier, and if you have breasts, one is likely larger than the other. That's why most bra straps are independently adjustable: to help support breasts of all shapes and sizes—even on the same body.

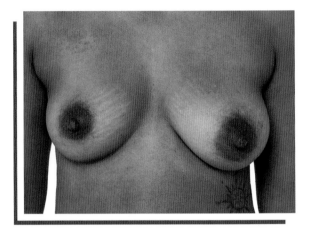

For people born with vaginas, it's not uncommon for breasts to grow at different speeds, especially in the first few years of puberty. Sometimes, the smaller breast "catches up," though not always. If you are concerned about how your breasts look in clothes, finding a bra with adjustable straps can help. Padded bras often have adjustable inserts, too, so you can either remove padding from the bigger side or add extra to the smaller side. (See page 89 for more on types of bras.)

> See your doctor if your breast size difference causes you concern. Uneven breasts are sometimes a sign of scoliosis, especially if the smaller breast has a smaller areola.

Can Big Breasts Affect Health?

There's no "good" or "bad" breast size or shape, but larger breasts tend to also be heavy. This can be quite the load for a body to bear, especially when they just showed up and you're still getting used to carrying around all the extra weight!

Big breasts can cause pain, skin rashes, headaches, and other health concerns—especially if not properly supported.

A great-fitting bra can help with a lot of heavy breast issues. While no specific exercise will lessen breast size, back and shoulder pain caused by heavy breasts might be improved by exercises designed to help improve posture and build up pectoral muscles as well as muscles in the back and shoulders, all of which help support heavy breasts behind the scenes.

While weight loss may cause some decrease in fat within the breasts, if a person already has a lean body shape, their large breasts are likely permanent and only reducible via medical intervention (see page 84 for more).

Underbreast Rashes

It's common, but not fun, for people with larger breasts to find an itchy, painful, and even smelly rash underneath their breasts at times. The skin in this dark, sometimes damp area doesn't have many opportunities to breathe, making it the perfect breeding ground for bacteria or fungus and sweat to mingle and cause trouble. A poorly fitting bra can add to the irritation (see page 89 for different types of bras to try).

Going braless (especially while sleeping) can help heal irritated skin in this area, as can blow-drying underneath the breast after a shower to make sure the area is bone dry (use the cool setting to avoid scorched skin). There are over-the-counter powders that can help heal and prevent underboob rashes as well.

Breast Reduction

A breast reduction is considered when neither a bra nor back exercises offer much relief from heavy breast pain. Breast reductions typically aren't performed until the surgeon is sure that breasts have stopped growing, preferably well into a person's twenties, but at least waiting until age eighteen. (The person in the following photo is a

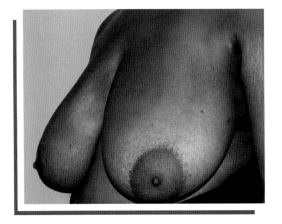

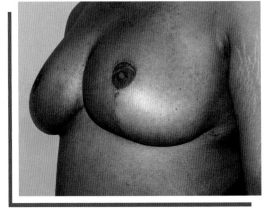

before breast reduction ⤵   ⤴ after breast reduction

twenty-two-year-old who had nearly two pounds per breast removed, which resolved their breast-related neck and back pain.) However, exceptions can be made for younger people suffering from serious breast-related health issues (like the ones mentioned on page 83), so talk to your doctor if your chest is causing you severe distress.

> For people who want to change the size of their chest to be larger (implants) or smaller (reduction or removal), whether for cosmetic reasons or to affirm their gender identity, it's a good idea to talk to a therapist before, during, and after the procedure to help unpack the "why" behind your desires, which may or may not be just about your chest.

Gender-Affirming Chests

Those who want to affirm their gender identity can get "top surgery," like breast implants, a breast reduction, or removal of almost all the breast tissue (as seen in the picture on the following page of a twenty-five-year-old). Bras, binders, and hormone therapies are other ways people can change the way their chest looks. See page 167 for more on gender and gender identity.

There are many reasons some people don't want to grow breasts, regardless of the genitalia they are born with. If the size of your chest makes you uncomfortable in any way (physically or emotionally), know that increasing exercise or limiting food is not a healthy or effective way to flatten your chest. It's important to talk about your feelings with either a doctor or a therapist to figure out a safe and satisfying solution. See page 197 for information on talk therapy and page 202 for more on eating disorders.

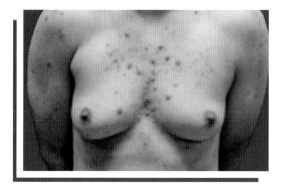

before breast tissue removal

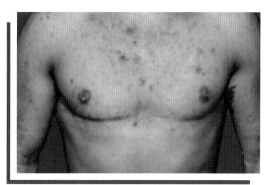

after breast tissue removal

Lumpy Breasts

While breast cancer in young adults is rare, it's common to have a few lumps in your breast tissue, which for many people feels lumpy in general. Checking your chest every month can help you to know what your breast tissue usually feels like—what could feel abnormally lumpy for someone else might just be normal for you. See page 86 for more on chest checking. If you feel some lumps, don't panic! There are many common noncancerous issues that can cause breast tissue lumps, including the following:

+ **Fibroadenomas.** Harmless, painless breast lumps made of solid tissue that typically feel hard and rubbery underneath the skin. They commonly show up around puberty.

- ✦ **Cysts.** Harmless, fluid-filled sacs in the breast that can be tender or painful to touch (especially around menstruation). They may develop as a result of hormonal changes.

- ✦ **Fibrocystic breasts.** A painful but harmless and very common recurring condition where breast cysts and swelling recur (come and go).

- ✦ **Menstrual cycle hormones.** Breasts can feel lumpier at different times of the month. To see if breast lumps are permanent or cycle-related, do a little extra examination and check your breasts twice in one month, both during menstruation and a week later, to see if any lumps felt during menstruation are still there. See page 87 for how to examine your breasts.

If you're still worried about any lumps you feel, it doesn't hurt to see your doctor and get checked out.

Time to Get Breast Aware! (And Chest Aware!)

Everybody can benefit from being "breast aware," which means you know what looks and feels normal for your chest and breasts. Early cancer detection makes a lot of difference in treatment outcomes—many breast cancers are first found by self-examination, especially in younger people! So the better you know your breast baseline, the easier you'll know if something feels or looks off, and the faster you can do something about it.

Everyone born with a vagina should check their chest on a regular basis—while a breast reduction or chest masculinization surgery can lower the risk of breast cancer, it's still possible.

People born with penises should inspect their chests, too—especially if they have a history of breast cancer in their biological family or have had feminizing gender-affirming hormone therapy.

Doing a Breast Check (or Chest Check)

It's easy (and kinda fun) to be breast aware.

First, give yourself a visual inspection to see how your breasts look. Study your breasts carefully in the mirror first with your hands down by your side, then with your hands clapped together and raised over your head. Do you see any changes in size, shape, or color since the last time you checked? Any new moles or freckles? Don't forget to peek at your underboob!

Then use your hands to physically inspect your breasts to see how they feel. Many find it easier to perform this exam in the shower or lying on their backs. Using the pads of your fingers, gently (but firmly) press all around each breast, one at a time, using these three direction techniques.

- **Clock.** Start underneath your armpit and move your fingers in small circles around your breast area, like a clock hand, working toward the nipple. Repeat for the other breast.

- **Pizza.** This time, start from your nipple and move your fingers out toward the edge of the breast, dividing sections like a pizza pie.

- **Sponge.** Next, slide your fingers up and down as if you're washing your breast with a sponge, covering the entire area.

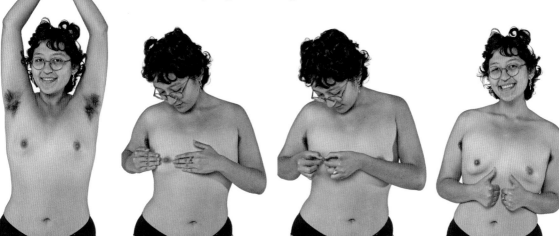

After you've checked for lumps, gently squeeze your areolas and nipples, and look for any discharge.

Try to do a breast check at the same time every month, ideally a few days after your period ends (if you menstruate). People who do not menstruate should pick a day of the month and stick to it. Keep notes on anything unusual you notice, either in a journal or a notes app. Your written breast health history will prove extremely helpful if you ever have an issue.

See your doctor if:

✦ You find swelling or a very firm lump in your breast that doesn't move when you press on it.

✦ You have any constant breast or nipple pain.

✦ You find a lump or swelling in your armpit.

✦ You find the same lump two months in a row.

✦ Your breast skin puckers or has other changes in color or texture.

✦ Your nipple suddenly inverts (see page 75 for more) or is leaking discharge.

If you feel a lump that you're certain didn't exist the month prior, it's common to panic and immediately start imagining the worst-case scenario. But try to relax—breast cancer in people born with vaginas under the age of thirty is possible but quite uncommon.

And while people born with penises *can* get breast cancer, it's rare but not impossible, so take a moment and check your chest, okay?

Congratulate yourself on putting your best chest forward!

If you're a person with limited mobility, giving yourself a thorough breast or chest exam may be difficult or impossible, but these exams are still an important part of your preventative care. Talk to your doctor about alternate strategies to help you care for your body and stay as healthy as possible.

Finding a Bra BFF

If you choose to wear a bra, it should behave like a good friend: uplifting and comfy to be with. And, like your friends, your bra should never make you feel uncomfortable or hurt you.

Finding the perfect bra involves trying out many different styles and fabrics. There are a few different ways to measure yourself for a bra, which can vary in accuracy depending upon the type of breasts you have. For example, pendulous breasts (as discussed on page 80) can be difficult to measure properly, and often it's best to do a bunch of try-on sessions to find the right style and size.

If you can, visit a store that offers professional measuring—it's usually free, and it helps give you a starting point. However you make it happen, if you decide to wear a bra, make sure to have fun figuring what type works for you!

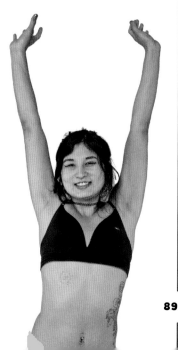

+ **Adaptive bras** are designed to support the breasts of people with limited mobility who may find it difficult or impossible to put on or keep on bras with hook-and-eye clasps or other traditional features. Adaptive bras come in hundreds of styles featuring many different adaptations, so a quick Internet search can usually find one to meet most needs.

+ **Training bras**, unlined and wireless, are often worn to help people get used to the idea of wearing bras or to offer coverage to prevent nipple friction in clothes.

- **Padded bras** have cushiony cup inserts to shape breasts and conceal nipples. These can be wireless or wired.

- **Underwire bras** have a wire that runs all along the base to give breasts extra lift and support. These can be padded or unpadded.

- **T-shirt bras** are built to be seamless, so the outline of the bra doesn't show beneath more formfitting tops. They can be padded or unpadded, wireless or wired.

- **Push-up bras** usually have underwire and padding and are designed to "perk up" breasts and create cleavage.

- **Bralettes** usually have no underwire or padding. They provide minimal support but are super comfy.

- **Bandeau bras** usually have no wiring, straps, or padding but do have extra support on the top and bottom bands to keep the bra in place. They tend to look like tube tops and are less confining than strapless bras, but also less defining.

- **Strapless bras** are . . . bras without straps. They're helpful when wearing tops that also don't have straps but where breast support is still needed.

- **Bra tape** is special, gentle-yet-strong tape designed to replace a bra in situations where more side and back skin shows, such as in an evening gown or swimsuit. Never substitute duct tape or even regular tape if it's not an adhesive specifically made for the breast, as the removal process can cause serious skin damage (and a lot of pain).

- **Minimizer bras** usually have more cup coverage than other bras and are meant to minimize the appearance of breasts.

- **Sports bras** are often made with thicker fabric and may have more hooks (or zippers) to compress breasts closer to the chest, creating a very tight and supportive fit that keeps breasts from bouncing too much during physical activity.

- **NO BRA!** If you decide that no bra is right for you, and you're comfortable going completely without one, that's fine, too. No one *has* to wear a bra, so feel free to be free!

Chest Binding

Chest binders, kinesiology tape, and compression tops are items people wear when they would like to minimize the appearance of their breast tissue beyond what a minimizing bra or sports bra can do, often to affirm their gender identity. If you can't get an actual binder or compression top made for the purposes of chest binding, never use plastic wrap, duct tape, or stretchy bandages as a substitute, as these household items aren't designed to be worn by a person and can cause breathing problems and serious injuries—even broken bones! Binders, specifically, can be very confining, and for your long-term health, they shouldn't be worn on very hot days, while exercising intensely, while sleeping, or for more than eight hours each day. Before putting your binder back on, make sure your skin is clean and dry and inspect your chest tissue every day for any sores or signs of infection. If something feels or looks off, stop wearing the binder immediately and see your doctor. People with asthma or other breathing concerns should see their doctor before beginning to chest bind.

bladders

&

bowels

We all do it, often multiple times a day. Peeing and pooping, of course! Indeed, everyone has a bladder and bowels, the function of which are urination and defecation—the proper medical terms for peeing and pooping.

Socially, we're brainwashed to think that emojis are the only type of poop that's okay to talk about. But that's not okay! Talking about stool is cool! Let's be free to discuss pee!

Feces (aka Poop)

Feces (the medical term for poop) are formed from the leftover waste after your bowels (the tube-shaped organ commonly known as your intestines) extract all the nutrients and most of the fluids from the foods you eat and the liquids you drink.

Feces are stored in the rectum, the last part of the large bowel. When you're ready to poop, formally known as defecating or having a bowel movement, feces are pushed out of the body through a puckered circle called the anal opening, or anus.

Everybody's natural bathroom habits are slightly different—and on average, people poop anywhere from three times a day to three times a week. If you go more than three times a day, you may have diarrhea, especially if it's runny. If you go fewer than three times a week, you may be constipated.

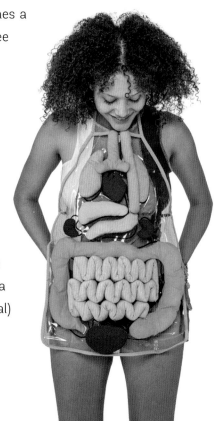

Poop Is Brown (Unless It's Not)

Healthy poop can be any shade of brown, as the process of digestion removes all the pigments from foods and a complex chemical called stercobilin gives poop its (usual) brown color. However, your poop can be different colors, whether due to illness or infection or just because some pigments aren't broken down by digestion, causing different-colored stools (poop).

Most non-brown poop isn't harmful, especially if the color doesn't show up frequently. Still, it's good to know what various colors of poop might mean.

- **Tan.** Infections can sometimes turn poop very light brown or tan. However, if you're taking medications, check with your doctor to see if light-colored stools might be a side effect.

- **Gray or off-white.** If your poop is frequently gray or off-white, it could be a sign that bile is not making its way into the stool, which can be due to liver trouble or a blockage in the bile duct. See your doctor.

- **Black or almost black.** Stomach blood can color poop black and might indicate bleeding from your stomach or small intestine. If you aren't taking iron supplements and haven't eaten foods that darken poop, like grape juice or black licorice, or taken medicines like Pepto-Bismol, see your doctor.

- **Green.** Surprise, surprise—green foods, like broccoli and spinach, can give your poop a greenish hue. Certain food dyes, like the ones in black jelly beans and grape Pedialyte, can cause green poop, too, as can iron supplements. Poop can also appear green if your bowels are moving faster than usual, like if you have a stomach bug.

- **Pink or red.** Beets, cranberries, or foods that might have red food coloring (like red frosting or candy) can turn your poop red or pink, but, occasionally, so can fresh blood. While seeing red on or in your stool when you wipe can be something common like menstrual blood (page 148) or hemorrhoids (page 97), see your doctor if this is persistent or worsening, especially if you haven't eaten anything that would cause red or pink poop.

Is Perfect Poop Possible?

There is no one picture-perfect poop because everyone's bowels work slightly differently. However, there are some questions to ask yourself as you snoop your stool:

+ **Is my poop well formed?** Healthy poop tends to look like a sausage link or hot dog. If it is runny (more liquid than solid), that's often a sign of diarrhea.

+ **Is my poop soft and smooth?** If you poke a healthy poop with a stick, a mark will usually be left. Hard and lumpy poop is often a sign of constipation.

+ **Is it easy for me to poop?** Healthy poop is usually comfortable to eliminate ("poop out"). If pooping hurts during or after, there may be a problem.

If you answered no to one or more of these questions, keep reading to see what might be causing your toilet troubles.

Runny Poop

Loose and runny poops are signs of diarrhea, and it usually means that something's off with your gut. Whether it's an infection, illness, food intolerance, something you ate, or medication you're taking, your food isn't staying in your colon long enough to form solid poops. Also, people who menstruate sometimes experience diarrhea as a complication of their cycle (see page 152 for more). Diarrhea ranges from sort of mushy to completely liquid, and elimination usually comes with an uncomfortable sense of urgency, often with pain (especially if you pass diarrhea frequently, which can cause your anus to be irritated).

> Healthy poops usually sink in the toilet water; floating poops may indicate you're suffering from excess gas or that your body may not be able to absorb fat properly.

Stuck Poop

Constipation is when poop has stayed in your colon for too long, often because there's not enough water in your body to help push it out. When you're constipated, your stool is hard and dry and usually difficult to eliminate without straining, discomfort, or pain. Common causes of constipation include dehydration, not eating enough fiber, stress, and some medicines. Also, people who menstruate sometimes experience constipation as a complication of their cycle (see page 152 for more). Holding in your poop instead of going when you feel the urge can cause constipation as well.

> Is your stool super shiny? Greasy, oily poops can be a sign that your body isn't able to properly absorb fat.

There's Blood When I Wipe!

Does it hurt when you poop or when you wipe after? Do you see bright red blood on your toilet paper or in the toilet (and you're not menstruating)? Do you feel pain, lumps, or bumps on your anus (it's totally okay to touch there, just wash your hands afterward)? You might have a hemorrhoid or an anal fissure.

Nearly half the population will, at some point in their life, suffer from hemorrhoids, which are swollen veins in the rectum or anus that can be painful and itchy and sometimes bleed. Hemorrhoids can be caused by pressure from constipation, diarrhea, sitting too long on the toilet, pregnancy, and pushing too hard when pooping.

External hemorrhoids hang out (literally) around your anus. You can see and feel these lumps, and they are usually painful or itchy to touch. You can't see internal hemorrhoids, and they are usually painless, but they are more likely to bleed.

Anal fissures can be mistaken for internal hemorrhoids, as both can cause anal bleeding, but fissures are more likely to be painful. One in ten people will experience anal fissures, which are tears inside the anus that can happen when the anal opening is stretched—by especially large or hard poop or if something is inserted inside of the anus.

While hemorrhoids or fissures are totally treatable, avoiding them in the first place is something to strive for by following the healthy poop suggestions on page 100.

If you're battling a burning bottom, a warm bath can help, as the heated water calms the hemorrhoids and fissures and helps them to heal. (If you don't have a tub, consider buying a specialized sitz bath, a small, shallow tub meant to soak and soothe the area.) When you soak, avoid bubble baths or other scented products, and stick to just water or gentle Epsom salt.

To help with pain and reduce inflammation, there are many over-the-counter ointments and pads made specifically for irritated anuses. But if the problem persists, see your doctor for a possible diagnosis and treatment options.

STI or Hemorrhoids?

If you find bumps and lumps around your anus and you're sexually active, there's a chance they might not be hemorrhoids but rather anal warts that are caused by a strain of the most common STI (sexually transmitted infection), the human papillomavirus (HPV). You cannot make this diagnosis on your own, so see your doctor immediately if you suspect anal warts. If caught early, they are treatable, but left untreated, they can spread and cause additional health complications.

Snoop on Your Poop

Doctors can analyze feces using stool testing. Stool testing can tell you things about your poop that you can't see with the naked eye—like if you have microscopic parasites or certain infections—and can help determine if you need to screen for other illnesses, including some cancers.

But you don't necessarily need to get your poop professionally analyzed when you can snoop your own poop! One look in the toilet after a bowel movement, and you can tell if you're drinking enough water, eating enough fiber (most of us aren't; see page 102 for fibrous foods), or ill. The color and texture can tell you a lot (as you learned earlier in this section). Also, if you have pinworms or other parasites (see the next section), your poop might show you wiggly evidence. But most of us just flush this treasure trove of health insights down the toilet without even looking at it.

> Wiping front to back (swooping from your genitals toward and beyond your anus) can help limit the spread of bacteria and avoid poop-covered labia or scrotums.

Poop Parasites

Is your bowel movement . . . moving? Even if you can't see anything wiggling in your poop, is your anus extremely itchy, especially at night? Or are you just really tired all the time and have symptoms of IBS like diarrhea, constipation, or stomach pain? There's a chance you may have joined the twelve million Americans infected with parasites. Parasites are transmitted by human or animal poop—you may have high-fived someone who didn't wash their hands after pooping and then accidentally touched your hand to your mouth, or your sweet pet may have licked your mouth after licking its butt. Some people get infected by eating raw fish—one person, after eating a lot of sushi, pooped out a tapeworm that was over five and a half feet long!

Once inside the body, many types of parasites like to live in our guts. Some worm parasites, like pinworms, exit the body at night to lay eggs around the anus. They can also exit the body when you poop—occasionally, you can see them in the toilet.

Not all parasites can be seen with the naked eye, so if you have any of the symptoms above and suspect you're infected, see your doctor as soon as possible so they can take a stool sample. It's important to treat a parasitic infection early because, left untreated, they can wreak havoc on your health. Fortunately, treatment for any type of intestinal parasite is pretty easy—usually a round of oral medicine kills the parasites inside of you so you can poop the remains out.

> Do you put the toilet lid down before flushing? If not, you may want to start, as research has found that infectious diseases can easily spread from "toilet plumes," which are the airborne bacteria from your poop that, upon flushing, can spread all over the bathroom— on the sink, up your nose, and even onto your toothbrush!

The Poop Improvement Plan

Having a pooping plan can really help to improve your poop and pooping experience. If you think you could be pooping better but don't know how, consider incorporating some of these tips and tricks. Your butt will thank you!

- **Schedule sacred pooping time.** Try to plan out your schedule so that you poop around the same time every day. The more you stick to a routine, the better your poops will be.

- **Go when ya gotta go.** Never wait for your scheduled pooping time if you have to go immediately. Holding in your poop instead of pooping when you feel the urge can eventually lead to chronic constipation because the longer the poop sits in your colon, the drier and bigger it becomes. It's then harder to eliminate and can be very painful upon exit, potentially causing an anal fissure (see page 97) and leading to other complications.

- **Don't take your time on the toilet.** Sitting on the toilet playing phone games may be fun for your brain, but it's bad for your butt. The toilet is not a toy; sit on it, do your business, and leave, or risk hemorrhoids from all the pressure (see page 97 for more on hemorrhoids).

- **Stop straining.** Gentle pushing to evacuate poop is fine, but straining runs the risk of causing bleeding, anal tears, and hemorrhoids.

- **Use a toilet stool.** Propping up your feet on a toilet stool (or a box) helps get your rectum in the best position for a smooth and comfortable poop.

> Physical movement helps your bowel movements. Daily exercise gets your body going and your poop flowing.

Limiting Laxatives

While occasional use of poop-producing products, such as any type of laxative (even the ones you buy at the drugstore), is reasonable, long-term use should be under a doctor's supervision. Exercising, eating healthy, and drinking lots of water will do the trick in most cases.

Sometimes long-term laxative use is necessary, but abuse is always a problem. People suffering from eating disorders often abuse laxatives, meaning they use the laxative more frequently and in larger amounts than recommended by their doctor or the product packaging. This can potentially lead to the body becoming dependent upon the product to go. See page 202 for more information on eating disorders and seeking help.

> If an adult unraveled their large intestine, it would be over five feet long! That sounds like a lot, but the small intestine is usually double or even triple that length—it's called "small" because of its width, not length.

Eat to Poop!
(Poop–Friendly Foods)

Sticking to whole and healthful foods can really help shape better poops. Fast food and other processed food that lacks vital nutrients and fiber are a main cause of crappier (ha!) poops. Some suggestions for what to ingest so poop can be at its best include:

- ✦ **Fiber.** Since your body can't digest fiber, eating fiber-filled foods helps to clean your colon and form healthy poops that are easy to eliminate. Most people don't eat enough fiber. Some foods full of fiber include bananas, nuts, oatmeal, apples, beans, and berries, as well as the hydrating foods listed on page 103. To get to the daily recommended grams of fiber for teenagers (25 to 31 grams), you can also take fiber supplements—just drink even more water than usual to make sure the fiber can make its way through your body.

- ✦ **Water.** All that fiber needs lots of water to help it move through your body, but you don't have to just drink it! Great ways to stay hydrated include water-filled foods like cucumbers, lettuce, and most fruits and vegetables. See page 103 for more.

- ✦ **Sorbitol-containing fruits.** Pears, prunes, apples, dates, and peaches contain not only a lot of fiber but also a carbohydrate called sorbitol, which helps the intestines retain water, keeping poop moving along.

- ✦ **Probiotic foods.** Fermented foods like yogurt, kimchi, miso, and pickles have live microorganisms called probiotics that can help with gut health and, thus, with healthy poops.

Some people's bowels just can't handle spicy foods without experiencing discomfort during bowel movements, as the mucosal lining of the anus is very sensitive to heat-producing spices, just like the mouth. Spicy food can also cause diarrhea. If you have this issue, consider limiting how often you eat spicy foods to avoid unnecessary suffering.

Avoiding Dehydration

Your bladder and bowels depend on a lot (A LOT) of fluids to run smoothly. Urine is almost entirely water (95 percent), and feces (poop) is 75 percent water.

When your body is well hydrated, meaning you consume enough water either from drinking or from the foods you eat, your urine is a light-yellow color with very little odor, and your bowels are more likely to make soft, smooth, heavy feces that are easy to pass.

When you're not well hydrated or are dehydrated, your urine has a higher concentration of body waste, making it darker colored and smellier. Your feces become drier, lumpier, and much harder to pass (see page 97 for more on constipation).

To help make healthy poop and pee, most people need to drink approximately half a gallon (1.8 liters) of fluids, ideally mostly water, each day—that's about the volume of a 2-liter bottle of soda. Of course, if you live in a hot climate or sweat a lot (from exercise or otherwise), you'll need more. Age, weight, and health status also figure into daily intake requirements.

Eat to Pee! (Hydration–Friendly Foods)

While drinking water is the best way to get your necessary 2 liters of fluid each day, sometimes you can supplement your water intake by eating your way to hydration! There are many vegetables and fruits that contain more than 90 percent water, and they can help achieve your hydration goals. An added bonus is that most of these foods contain a lot of fiber, which helps with poop!

- ✦ Cucumbers
- ✦ Radishes
- ✦ Tomatoes
- ✦ Cauliflower
- ✦ Mushrooms

- ✦ Lettuce
- ✦ Cantaloupe
- ✦ Cabbage
- ✦ Strawberries
- ✦ Celery

- ✦ Watermelon
- ✦ Spinach
- ✦ Squash
- ✦ Pickles

CAUTION: Food sensitivities and allergies should be taken very seriously when trying products, foods, and recipes mentioned in this manual. If you are allergic or think you might be sensitive to anything suggested, don't try it! Food allergies also apply to what you put on your skin. For example, if your throat tingles when you drink coconut water, don't use coconut oil as an emollient (as suggested on page 16). Or if you have an oat allergy, avoid the oatmeal-honey scrub suggested on page 15. When in doubt, leave it out!

Urine (aka Pee)

Urine (the medical term for pee) is a mixture of excess water and the waste your kidneys filter from your body's blood.

Urine is stored in the bladder, a stretchy, bag-like organ that can hold up to 16 ounces for a few hours at a time before you have to urinate.

When you pee, urine exits your body through the urethra, the tube that connects your bladder to your genitals. The opening to the urethra in people with vaginas is between the clitoris and the vaginal opening. For people with penises, the urethral opening is usually in the center of the head of the penis and is also used to ejaculate semen (more on that on page 140).

Most people urinate up to seven times each day. See your doctor if you're urinating more frequently or if you're urinating fewer than two times a day, as this could be a sign of an underlying medical issue.

> A urologist is a type of doctor who helps you care for your urinary system, and a gastroenterologist helps you care for your digestive system.

Pee Is Yellow (Unless It's Not)

Healthy urine is usually shaded yellow because of urobilin, a yellow chemical the body produces while creating waste. The more water you drink, the more diluted the urobilin is in your urine, making it a lighter shade of yellow. So, healthy urine is a very pale yellow because your body is properly hydrated.

If you don't consume enough water, you're likely dehydrated, so the urobilin in your urine will be more concentrated, turning your pee a darker shade of yellow or even brownish.

Temporarily peeing the rainbow tends to be harmless and likely results from what you've recently had to eat or drink. However, there are some hues that you should see your doctor about, especially if you don't think you're eating or drinking anything to cause it.

+ **Neon orange or yellow** (super-bright) pee can be caused by certain medicines or vitamins.

+ **Green** could be from eating asparagus, vitamins, or food coloring, or it could be from an infection, especially if it's paired with pain while peeing.

+ **Pink** can come from the pigment in beets, rhubarb, and some berries. When people eat beets and pee pink, it's called beeturia. Pink can also be a sign of blood in your urine (see next bullet point).

+ **Red** urine could indicate blood in your urine, which generally is a sign of an infection. If you are not on your period (when blood usually drips into the toilet while urinating) and haven't eaten beets, berries, or rhubarb recently, see your doctor to rule out any concerns.

+ **Dark orange-brown** urine is a sign of serious dehydration or a liver problem, especially if paired with light-colored poops or yellowed eyes. See your doctor.

+ **Black** urine can happen to people who are sick with malaria or melanoma. See your doctor.

Aside from color, healthy urine should also be:

+ **Transparent.** While the color of urine can change, healthy pee shouldn't be cloudy, milky, or murky, as that's a sign that you may have an infection or an illness such as kidney stones (see page 109 for more).

+ **Mostly particle-free.** While it's normal to have a few bits of mucus or tissue in your urine, if you're noticing a lot of particles in your pee, it could be a sign that something's off.

+ **Flat, not foamy.** Having fizzy, bubbly, or foamy urine is not always abnormal—sometimes it happens when your pee stream is very strong, especially first thing in the morning, after you've held your urine for a long time. However, it can also be a sign of dehydration, and foamy urine can sometimes signify kidney issues or diabetes.

+ **Not (super) stinky.** Healthy urine generally has some smell, but if you're properly hydrated, it shouldn't be strong. There are a few reasons your urine might stink. Some people find their pee smells foul after consuming certain medicines or vitamins; drinks like beer, coffee, and soda; and foods like garlic, onions, fish, and asparagus. An infection can also cause smelly urine, so if you notice an odor that doesn't improve with drinking more fluids or changing your eating habits, you might want to see your doctor.

If you don't have a penis and want to pee standing up—especially when there's no clean restroom around where you can sit and pee, there are special pee funnels available that make it much easier to go on the go!

See What's in Your Pee

Urine is like your BFF—it knows things about you that no one else does. When something feels or looks off, you can pee in a cup, and doctors can analyze your urine through a process called urinalysis. Similar to stool (poop) testing (see page 98), urinalysis is a series of visual and chemical pee tests that can tell all kinds of things about you based on the waste your kidneys filter out of your blood and into your pee, such as your eating habits, certain illnesses and infections you might have, what drugs or medicines you take, and more. Some types of urinalysis you can do at home yourself, like pregnancy and urinary tract infection tests. However, always call your doctor if you get a positive result or if symptoms persist with a negative result.

Bed-Wetting Is Not Uncommon!

If you're wetting the bed, you aren't alone—nighttime control is the last form of urinary control people develop, and it takes longer for some, so bed-wetting may be normal for your body.

People of all ages can be bed-wetters. In fact, 1 in every 50 teenagers suffers from nocturnal enuresis, the fancy term for accidental (involuntary) urination while sleeping. (Don't confuse bed-wetting with "wet dreams," which is when semen or other orgasmic fluids are released while sleeping, and which you can read more about on page 141.)

There are many reasons you might wet the bed. Drinking too much water before bedtime is one, and sleeping disorders, medications, illnesses, infections (like a UTI, page 108), and even stress can affect your ability to hold your urine while sleeping, too. Some people are just very deep sleepers, and their bodies can't wake them up to walk to the bathroom. It can be hereditary—people with a birth parent who wet the bed into later childhood or the teen years are more likely to do so themselves. Bed-wetting usually goes away with time, but if this is happening to you, talk to your doctor, as they can help you pinpoint your pee problem and find a solution, especially if you are unable to hold your urine during the day.

> Sometimes urinary incontinence can be caused by constipation when backed-up feces press on the bladder. See page 97 for more on constipation.

Painful Pee

It should never hurt or be uncomfortable to pee—any sort of pain, burning, stinging, pressure, or itching before, during, or after peeing is a sign that something's off.

You might feel the urge to pee all the time, even if you just went to the bathroom and don't have any urine stored in your bladder. The urine you pass might also be cloudy or smell worse than usual.

This discomfort is usually caused by a urinary tract infection (UTI for short). Your bladder, kidneys, urethra, and ureters are all part of the urinary tract. Sometimes a certain type of bacteria (or occasionally a fungus or virus) makes its way into the urinary tract, causing it to become irritated or inflamed.

UTIs are extremely common and can happen to anyone, though people with vaginas are more vulnerable, as their urethras are much shorter, making it easier to get infected.

For years, mainstream advice about preventing UTIs revolved around always wiping front to back, never holding your pee, and urinating immediately after sexual activity. However, while it can't hurt to try these tactics, recent guidelines put out by the American Urological Association suggest that more than likely, if you get UTIs often it's not because of something you are doing or not doing. So don't blame yourself!

Drinking enough water might help prevent UTIs (and is just good for you in general). See page 103 for tips on getting enough water.

Most UTIs stay in the bladder and urethra, but they can spread if left untreated. Untreated UTIs can cause a more serious kidney infection, leading to complications and permanent damage. In very rare cases, an untreated UTI can cause a fatal blood infection. So see your doctor if you think you have a UTI!

There can be other causes of urinary tract irritation and discomfort that are not due to an infection. Things you eat and drink can be irritating—some find that eliminating certain foods and beverages, such as coffee, soda, spicy foods, citrus, and anything sugary, can help. Eliminating all douches, perfumed soaps, lotions, or sprays in the genital area can reduce irritation as well. Spermicides and lubricants can also often cause irritation. See your doctor if you're dealing with painful pee that doesn't go away after a day or two or if the pain returns. Your doctor can determine exactly what you need to help the issue go away while ensuring it's not something more serious like a sexually transmitted infection (see page 185) or another medical problem.

Kidney Stones

Kidney stones are on the rise in young adults. When you don't hydrate your body adequately (through water or fruits and vegetables), sometimes the waste materials and minerals that your kidneys filter out of your body aren't able to stay dissolved in your urine. When that happens, the waste and minerals may form crystals in the kidneys that bind together to create small, solid masses called kidney stones.

While some kidney stones stay in the kidney, where they're harmless, others travel and make their way to the ureter (the tube that connects your kidney to your bladder). That's when they start to cause pain. When stones are small enough to pass through the ureter to the bladder, they can usually exit your body when you pee. However, bigger stones cannot pass easily and may block urine drainage. This can lead to pain (lots of pain!) in your back or side, blood in your urine, nausea, and vomiting.

While drinking lots of water can help you avoid kidney stones, dehydration isn't the only cause. Getting stones can also be hereditary, which is why when you first get a kidney stone, especially as a kid or young adult, often your doctor will want to find out your family history and what your health habits are, in order to try to prevent future episodes.

If you suspect a stone, keep drinking water and see your doctor.

Burps and Farts

We all pass gas and a lot of it, too: up to twenty-five times each day. When you pass gas from your mouth, that's called belching, commonly known as burping. When you pass gas from your anus, that's called flatulence, widely known as farting.

Burping and farting are important bodily functions; when you burp or fart, you release excess gas and air from the body that would otherwise cause you pain and discomfort (keep reading for more on bloating). In a perfect society, farting and burping would be as normal and shame-free as sneezing. So let 'er rip . . . for your health!

Burps mostly come from air that is swallowed. Every time you eat, drink, laugh, talk, and even sleep (especially if you snore), you're swallowing excess air that makes its way to your esophagus or stomach, and it must come out. Sometimes your burps pick up the odor of what you've eaten or drunk recently—that's totally normal.

While some farts come from swallowed air that makes its way into the intestines, most are actually from gases your body produces as it digests the foods you eat. That's why some foods, like beans, cause more flatulence. However, unlike burps, farts usually don't smell like food. Many farts are odorless, despite their reputation. Stinky farts, however, are also normal.

Almost all foods cause the body to produce gas, but some foods are more burp-and-fart fuel than others. Cabbage, broccoli, beans, and lentils are common high-gas culprits, but your body may be different and have different toot triggers.

If you find yourself constantly burping or farting, look at your eating and drinking habits first.

Drinking carbonated drinks like soda can cause you to burp a lot—the only way most of the swallowed air from the fizzy drink can be released is by burping. That's why it's more common to burp after drinking a bottle of sparkling water than it is after you drink a glass of tap water. Chewing gum, talking while eating, drinking from a straw, or eating too quickly causes you to swallow more air as well.

If eating or burping causes a burning feeling in your throat, chest, or neck during or afterward, you may be suffering from acid reflux, the main symptom of which is heartburn. Heartburn after eating is very common in teens.

Sometimes this discomfort is due to eating habits, but some people just get more acid reflux than others. If there's post-eating pain in your throat or chest more than once a week or so, see your doctor to figure out what's going on and how to help.

> If you find yourself unable to pass gas in either direction, see your doctor. Some people suffer from no-burp syndrome, where they are physically unable to burp and must seek treatment to relieve the discomfort. Being unable to fart for an extended period of time, accompanied by belly pain or vomiting, can actually be a sign that something serious is wrong, like a bowel obstruction.

Balloon Belly (Bloating)

Does your belly ever feel bloated, like an overfilled balloon? Trapped gas is one of the main reasons people become bloated, as is fluid retention, constipation, eating a large amount of food, taking fiber supplements, and some food intolerances. Stress can also cause bloating, as can some illnesses. People who menstruate may find that they bloat at certain times of their cycle, generally due to fluid retention.

Most bloating is temporary, and helping the trapped air escape your ballooned belly by burping or farting can deflate the situation (see page 110 for more on burps and farts). Hydration (page 103), exercise, stomach massage, and pooping can help, too.

If you're bloated for more than a day or two in a row, or your bloating seems to be getting worse, see your doctor.

At first, when you're improving your eating and exercise habits, you might think your poop and bloating problems are getting worse, but they're not! Your body is just adjusting to your new normal of healthy living, and you may even retain water and pass more gas at first as your body adjusts. It can take a few weeks for everything to normalize, so while you're in the transition phase, don't be surprised if you find yourself in the bathroom more than usual.

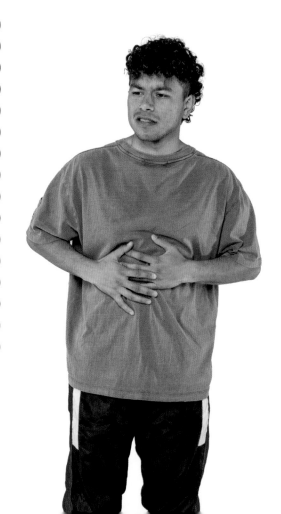

Digestion Difficulties

Some find certain foods difficult or impossible to comfortably digest—causing more-than-usual levels of burping, farting, and bloating, as well as other bathroom problems like diarrhea, constipation, and even rectal bleeding and severe allergic reactions. Dairy (animal milk and milk products like cheese and yogurt) and gluten (grains like wheat and rye) are common culprits for digestive drama, but a person can have problems digesting all kinds of ingredients, from caffeine to sugar to eggs to nuts.

If you're suffering from frequent bloating and problematic poops, consider keeping a bathroom journal to log information for yourself and your doctor. For a week or two, write down everything you eat and drink (including medication), as well as the time, appearance, and smell of each pee and poop. If there's any pain or discomfort before, during, or after using the bathroom, write that down, too, and look back at what you recently ate to see if you can spot the cause. You might be surprised by the patterns you see!

For example, if you drink a milkshake and have pain the next time you poop, that could be a sign that dairy is a cause for concern. If your stomach painfully bloats after you eat a bowl of pasta, gluten might not be great for your body. Being able to show your doctor your bathroom journal and your body's reaction to eating certain foods helps you advocate for yourself, your health, and your healing. Your doctor can help you determine if you're dealing with a food allergy, intolerance, or sensitivity—all issues that look similar but require different treatments. Your doctor can also try to rule out more complicated digestive problems or refer you to a specialist (ideally a gastroenterologist) who can screen for and possibly diagnose a more serious digestive issue, like the next two discussed.

> Healthy poops usually don't resemble what you've eaten, except for the occasional indigestible food like corn or seeds. If you're chewing your food well and still regularly seeing chunks of it in your poop, see your doctor, as it might be a sign of a more serious digestion-related condition, especially if you have other symptoms.

Irritable Bowel Syndrome (IBS)

Affecting about 1 out of every 6 people in North America, IBS is a disorder of the gastrointestinal tract that causes uncomfortable and often unpredictable symptoms like bloating, abdominal pain, and sometimes feeling worse after eating, and long-term constipation, diarrhea, or a combination of both. In addition, stress and certain foods (especially dairy) may worsen IBS symptoms. While there's no specific test available yet to diagnose IBS, you should still see your doctor if you have symptoms. They can ask you questions, check your overall health, and screen for other digestive issues like IBD.

Inflammatory Bowel Disease (IBD)

Diseases that cause intestinal inflammation are on the rise, including Crohn's disease and ulcerative colitis, which are types of inflammatory bowel disease (IBD). IBD symptoms can be similar but are usually more severe than those of IBS and may include vomiting, lack of appetite, weight loss, fever, anemia, and rectal bleeding. It is possible to simultaneously have both IBS and IBD. If diagnosed, there are therapies and medications that can be helpful with some IBD, so see your doctor if you have any of these symptoms. They can run various tests to figure out what's going on, whether it's IBD or another concern.

Celiac Disease

Gluten is a protein found in foods made from wheat, barley, and rye, and celiac disease is an autoimmune disorder that causes the immune system to attack the body when gluten is consumed. When gluten is eaten by someone with celiac disease, even in small amounts, that person may experience symptoms like abdominal pain, bloating, constipation, diarrhea, nausea, and fatigue. Younger people diagnosed with celiac disease might experience delayed puberty and slowed growth. Currently, the only treatment is strict avoidance of gluten. This can be difficult, as it can be a surprise ingredient in many things, from jelly beans to hot dogs. See your doctor for a possible diagnosis and for support (like a referral to a registered dietitian to learn how to follow a gluten-free diet), as celiac disease can cause other health issues if left untreated.

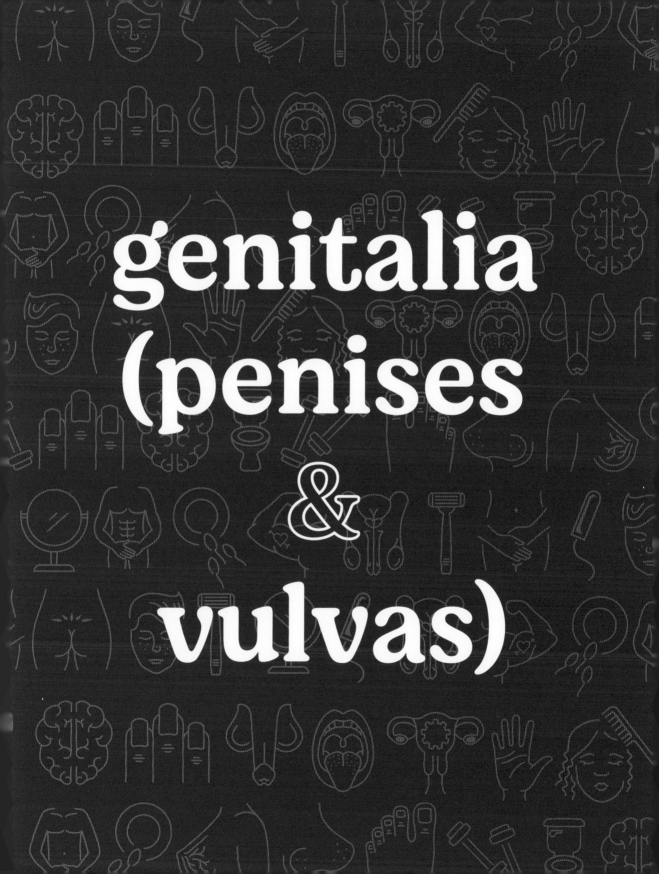

genitalia (penises & vulvas)

Most styles of underwear completely cover up your genitalia, which are located between your legs. Like fingerprints, no two are the same—everyone's genitalia are one of a kind, with different shapes, colors, lengths, textures, and smells—and that's a great thing!

Genitalia have three main functions:

+ Urination (peeing)

+ Pleasure (yay)

+ Reproduction (making new humans)

It's important to be able to understand and talk comfortably about what a lot of us are used to calling "down there"—especially your own. While there's no one "normal" penis or vulva, and all genitalia are different, there are important aspects of genitalia health that everyone should know. That's where this section of the manual comes in—to give you the language and the information you need to love your body, have no shame, and get the help you need when you need it!

Internal & External Genitalia

Genitalia are more complicated than you might think and are made up of *many* organs, both external (what you can see) and internal (inside your body).

External genitalia (like the photos you'll see in this section) are what most of us think of when we hear the word "genitals." Most people's external genitalia are either a vulva (which you might be calling a vagina) or a penis and scrotum, but there is a super diverse spectrum of genitalia. Keep reading for more on external genitalia and turn to page 123 for information on the many different appearances of genitalia.

Internal genitalia involve lots of organs, including the body's primary reproductive organs. (More on reproduction on page 171.) Testicles are the primary reproductive organs of people born with penises. They are usually found inside the scrotum.

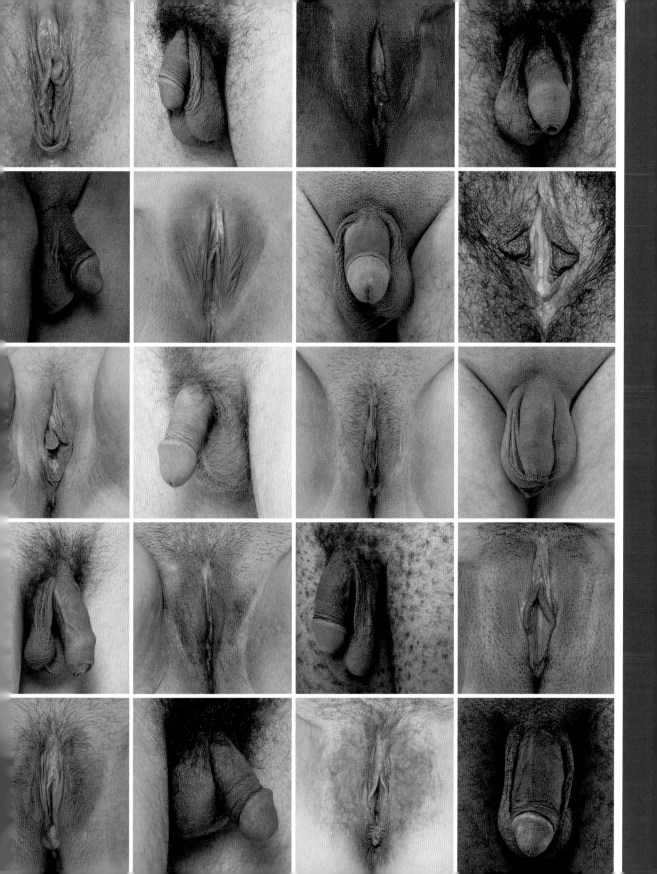

Ovaries are the primary reproductive organs of people born with vaginas. They usually are found inside the body on each side of the uterus (which is in the lower abdomen). People with intersex variations can have any combination of internal and external genitalia (more on intersex variations on page 165).

location of testicles ⟋   location of ovaries ⟍

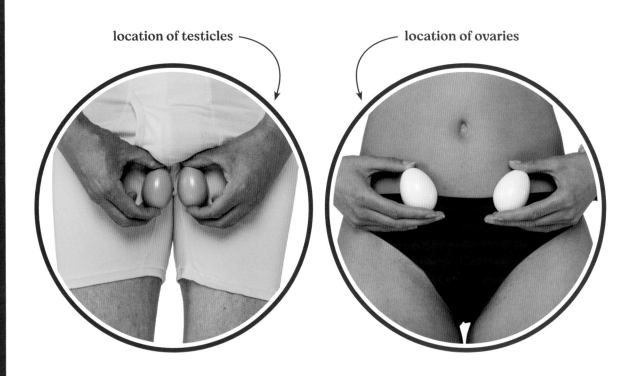

Many people refer to the vulva as a vagina, but they're actually two separate body parts. The vagina is part of your internal genitalia. More on vaginas starts on page 146!

In the womb, testicles and ovaries both develop from the same tissue, and even once fully formed they have a lot in common. Both come in pairs and are oval-shaped, and when they activate at puberty, they start producing the same key hormones to help the body mature, just in very different amounts—see page 164 for more on hormones.

Genitalia Grows for Years!

All of the genitalia photographed for this manual belong to adult bodies. So if you're searching for one in this manual that looks exactly like or similar to yours, remember that you might have a few more years to go before your genitals are fully matured. Genitalia can grow and change for many years, so don't be shocked if the genitalia you have in high school looks different when you're twenty-one.

Colorful Crotches

Know that whatever color your genitalia are naturally is normal—there's no one "right" color. Crotches are meant to be colorful! During puberty, hormones usually produce additional melanin, and nearly everyone experiences some level of skin darkening around the external genitalia. Healthy genitalia can be purple, brown, gray, red, pink, peach, burgundy, black . . . or a combination of all these colors. However, if you notice new discolorations like moles or lighter splotches, or if new colorations are paired with lumps, pain, or swelling, see your doctor.

Good–Feeling Genitalia

Your genitalia should always feel good—ideally great! Whether you're sitting, standing, exercising, or touching yourself for hygiene, curiosity, or pleasure (or a combination of the three), it is not healthy to feel any pain, itching, burning, stinging, or other unpleasant sensation in or around your penis, testicles, or vulva. If your genitalia don't feel good and you aren't sexually active, it is likely something minor is causing discomfort. Itchy genitalia could be a fungal infection like jock itch (see page 42), yeast (page 43 for everyone and page 158 specifically for vaginal yeast infections), or another type of infection. Or it could be genital psoriasis or eczema (page 40). If you are sexually active, see your doctor, as it could be something more serious, like a sexually transmitted infection, or STI (page 185). And sometimes it's something else that's not super serious but probably needs to be checked out, like a penile adhesion (page 132) or a Bartholin's cyst (page 144).

Good-Smelling Genitalia

Naturally, everyone's genitalia have some sort of smell (and it's not roses). The standard scent of your genitalia can be slightly cheesy, somewhat sweet, musky, acidic, or a combination of various scents. You can have a very strong smell . . . or almost no smell at all. Your hormones, the food you eat, and even your underwear can affect your personal *eau de you.*

Getting familiar with your unique odors can help you know when something's not right. Sniffing out your signature scent is simple—at different times of the day, just use your fingers to gently explore your genitalia and then smell your fingers. (It's a good idea to wash your hands both before and after.) A good baseline is what you smell like an hour or two after bathing, with no products applied to your body. That's when there's just enough aroma for you to know what you're supposed to smell like without sweat or built-up body odor masking it.

Once you become aware of your body's bouquet, if you feel it's altered for the worse, there are a few reasons to consider:

✦ **Are you cleaning your genitalia properly and often?** The longer genital grime stays on your body, the stronger the odor becomes. At least once a day, rinse your genitalia with warm water. If things are especially icky or you've missed a couple of cleanings, you can use a little soap meant for sensitive skin, gently rubbing the area with your fingers to rid it of the smell-causing ingredients. Be careful not to get soap up your urethra or in your vagina (if you have one). See page 13 for more tips on how to properly clean your genitalia folds as well as the rest of your body.

✦ **Is your underwear clean?** Even if it looks okay, tiny amounts of genital discharge, urine, and poop can accumulate throughout the day. If this stuff makes its way onto your genitalia, you could smell, feel sticky and itchy, or even get an infection. So change your underwear at least once daily!

✦ **Do you have an infection?** Many types of infections have an odor as a side effect, like bacterial vaginosis for people with vaginas (see page 159) and balanitis for people with penises (page 132). Jock itch can also cause odor in all people (page 42), as can some STIs (page 185). Check those pages and read about the different types of infections, and if you think you have one, see your doctor, as they can help you get it under control with the proper treatment if needed.

Don't Dare to Compare Genitalia!

Ever heard the phrase "comparison is the thief of joy"? It's so hard not to measure ourselves against others, especially when it comes to sensitive issues like how our genitalia look. But the game of constant comparing and contrasting is unwinnable, and not even fun to play. There will always be someone who has something you crave, whether it's their hair color or their clear skin, their penis width or their labia color. But guess what? The person with the traits you covet is likely dealing with their own insecurities, possibly with the same body parts that you think are perfection. Break the cycle of comparison and take back your joy!

Don't Let Others Compare You, Either

Bottom line about your bottom parts: if someone says something rude or hurtful about the size, shape, or smell of your genitalia, they are the ones with the problem, not you. Usually people are rude about others' bodies because they're insecure themselves. Learn to accept and love yourself just as you are and encourage those in your life to do the same. Consider that someone might be misguided and not completely cruel when they say something problematic, like comparing your body parts to the (probably airbrushed) people on their computer screens, and don't take it personally. You can break the cycle of bodily shame by showing them this manual for an accurate anatomy lesson to help them realize they have been wrong all along!

Considering Penis or Labia Surgery? Read This!

Thank goodness that genital surgeries and similar procedures are available to help so many people, like those who are born with genitalia variations that cause health complications, people seeking gender-affirming care, and people whose genitals are injured in a serious car accident (which causes genitalia trauma more often than you might think).

But while procedures like these can be lifesaving for people who are born with or acquire medical complications that affect their genitalia, studies have shown that most people seeking surgeries like penile enlargement or labiaplasty (to reduce labia size) have perfectly normal and healthy functioning genitalia. In these cases, the problems they're trying to surgically solve aren't originating from their physical bodies but from the pressure for "perfection" from the outside world.

Pornography, misinformation (or lack of information), cruel people, or a combination of all three and more can really mess with self-esteem and cause unrealistic expectations about what is considered average or physically attractive, and genitalia are no exception. When your erect penis is "just" four inches (which is normal) or your labia are dark and "flappy" (also normal), society can make you feel like your body is unlovable and gross, and that's not right. Or true!

Your body deserves to exist and be loved just as it is, but there's a widespread rumor ruining self-esteem nationwide that the "best" penises should be arm-shaped and massive, and that "pretty" vulvas should be small, a single color, and symmetrical. News flash: most genitalia don't naturally look that way, so it's no wonder that plastic surgery on genitalia has been increasing in popularity.

Sometimes scientific studies on "average" genitalia size don't help, either—many only measure a few dozen people, or study one ethnicity, or leave out specific demographics that the researchers felt would skew the data. Even studies that strive for diversity may not represent the full spectrum of humanity because not everyone is comfortable or capable of participating in such a personal study, even when it's anonymous.

None of this matters anyway, because scrotums aren't designed to be scrutinized! Labia don't deserve a label! (There are so many more positivity puns that could be made, but just know that you're great as you are.) Not only are penile enlargement and labiaplasty expensive—upwards of five thousand dollars and often much more—but also people who undergo these surgeries sometimes lose pleasurable sensation after surgery. And generally speaking, no amount of plastic surgery can totally get rid of bodily shame—there will always be something else to feel bad about if you don't work on self-acceptance from the inside out.

Talk therapy can really help you sort out feelings about your genitalia (and other issues that might be making you feel insecure or uncomfortable), so check out the suggestions on page 197. And if you are experiencing genital dysfunction or pain, like if your labia are so long that it hurts to sit down, or if you have erectile dysfunction (page 142), do talk to your doctor, as there are many legit reasons you may need genitalia surgery—just don't let senseless societal ideals be one of them.

Perineums

The sensitive area between your anus and the bottom of your genitals is called the perineum. Everybody's perineum stretches to help with pooping and peeing. It is also an erogenous zone and can feel very good to touch. When you wash your genitalia (which should be daily) and when you wipe yourself after using the bathroom, don't forget to clean your perineum, too, to avoid odor and potential infection.

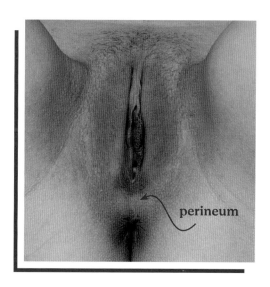

perineum

What's This White Stuff?

There's a substance that's specific to genitalia that can contribute to smell if not washed off often enough: smegma. Smegma is a whitish, cottage-cheese-looking secretion found in the folds of genital skin, like on the tip and under the foreskin of penises, in labial folds, and around the clitoris of vulvas. Don't stress if you see it! It's a natural, normal combination of bodily fluids (like oils, urine, and sweat) and dead skin cells that is lubricating for all genitalia and can even help break up penile adhesions (see page 132). But if smegma stays on your body for too long, it can build up and become stinky and sticky, causing irritation and inflammation on the surrounding skin. So, if you see a whole lot of smegma on your genitalia, try to bathe more often or more carefully (see page 10 for bathing tips).

smegma

Sometimes the way this manual describes genitalia may not exactly fit how your body parts look or feel, and that's nothing to be ashamed of! Remember: every body is different, and some require a little more personalized care. See your doctor and share what's going on "down there" so that you can best take care of yourself and stay as healthy as possible.

Genital Lumps and Bumps

Lumps or bumps on genitalia are usually just pimples (see page 19), razor burn (page 24), or ingrown hairs (page 65). Sometimes you can even get molluscum contagiosum on your genitalia, too (page 27). However, there are a few types of lumps and bumps that specifically show up on your genitalia.

Two scary-looking (at first) but not life-threatening genital lumps and bumps that have nothing to do with sexual activity include pearly penile papules (page 131) and Bartholin's cysts (page 144).

If you are or have been sexually active, itchiness, lumps, or bumps could be a sign of an STI that you need to tell your doctor about, like genital warts or herpes.

+ **Genital warts.** Cauliflower-like painless bumps that can be found on the penis, vulva, or anus that are caused by the human papillomavirus (HPV). Because all it takes to contract HPV is skin-to-skin contact with an infected part of the body, most sexually active people get it. Talk to your doctor about whether or not you're eligible for the HPV vaccine, which can help prevent genital warts and other HPV-related problems, such as cancer. If you think you have genital warts, see your doctor, who can often help lessen the visible lesions and treat or prevent additional HPV complications.

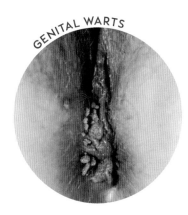
GENITAL WARTS

+ **Genital herpes.** Painful and itchy blisters or sores found on and around the vulva, penis, scrotum, anus, face, and in the throat and vaginal canal may be caused by the herpes simplex virus 2 (HSV-2). It's easy to catch HSV-2 through skin-to-skin contact, which is why more than 10 percent of people are infected. Despite looking similar, genital herpes is not

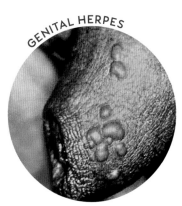
GENITAL HERPES

the same as the oral fever blisters and cold sores caused by herpes simplex virus 1 (see page 18 for more). See your doctor for diagnosis and treatment.

If your doctor does confirm an STI, it's important to find out if your past and current sexual partners should get tested, too. There is no cure for genital warts or herpes, but medication can help prevent complications and make outbreaks fewer and farther between.

> Testicles sometimes develop unexpected lumps, too! See page 135 for how to perform a testicular self-exam.

And no matter what, *never* pop bumps in or around your genitalia, as this can cause scarring and infection, not to mention a whole lot of pain. It's important to see your doctor if your bumps or discomfort persist—especially if you're sexually active.

> Although the anus is *near* the genitalia and has some similarities to genitalia, namely that touching it can bring pleasure, the anus is actually part of the digestive system. (More on butts and bowels starting on page 94).

Penises

The penis is a single organ with a few different parts. The visible parts (what you can see) include:

+ **The shaft.** The "main," tube-shaped part of the penis. The shaft is the part of the penis that can become erect (see page 137). While always cylindrical, the shaft can be thick, thin, curved left, pointed up . . . whatever your shaft looks like naturally is great. Internally, the shaft is connected to the penile root, which is how the penis attaches to the body.

- **The glans.** The rounded head of the penis, also known as the tip. It's extremely sensitive to touch.

- **The corona.** The rounded ridge around the base of the glans.

} Uncircumcised and circumcised penises have different hygiene routines—see page 13 for more. }

- **The foreskin (optional).** If you were born with a penis, you either have or once had a foreskin. Like a baseball helmet on your head, the foreskin protects the glans, covering it unless it is pulled back or removed. Sometimes the foreskin is surgically removed in a procedure called circumcision. Parents and guardians may circumcise a child shortly after birth for religious or cultural reasons. Occasionally, foreskins are removed later in life due to medical conditions. Both circumcised and uncircumcised penises are healthy and normal as long as there is no pain or difficulty urinating or ejaculating.

} Vulvas also have a fold of skin similar to a foreskin—the clitoral hood (see page 145). }

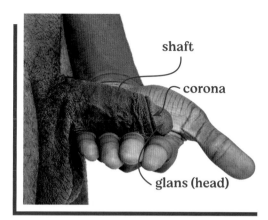

This person has been circumcised.

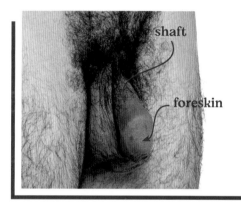

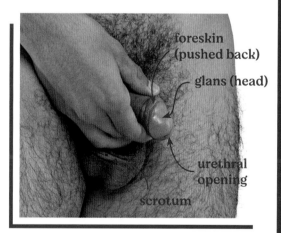

The person in these two pictures has not been circumcised, so their foreskin is intact. Uncircumcised people need to pull their foreskin back in order to see the glans.

+ **The frenulum.** The raised ridge of tissue that connects the underside of the shaft to the glans. In uncircumcised penises, the frenulum also connects the foreskin to the glans (see page 129 for more on the foreskin). The area around the frenulum is a powerful erogenous zone, meaning it's very sensitive to touch (in a good way).

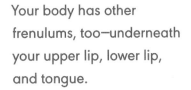

Your body has other frenulums, too—underneath your upper lip, lower lip, and tongue.

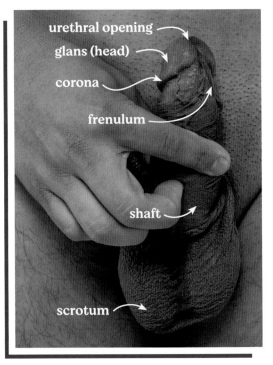

This person is uncircumcised and is pulling their foreskin back.

+ **The urethral opening.** A slit in the penis, usually in the center of the head (glans), that is the opening to the urethra. The urethra is the tube through which urine and semen exit the body.

In the United States, around 1 out of every 250 people born with penises has a urethral opening that is not in the center of the glans and instead can be found anywhere else on the penis. This is known as hypospadias, and depending upon the location of the urethral opening, people with hypospadias might find it more comfortable to urinate sitting down and sometimes can have painful erections and fertility problems. Often hypospadias is identified in infancy, but if you are concerned that your urethral opening is not in the center of your glans, see your doctor.

Almost half of people born with penises have little bumps called pearly penile papules (shown in this photo) on their corona. Aside from being a tongue twister, pearly penile papules don't hurt and aren't any reason for worry. They usually show up during puberty for unknown reasons and aren't caused by poor hygiene or sexually transmitted infections—people with perfectly healthy penises get PPP, too. (See page 127 for info on other bumps that might appear elsewhere on your penis.)

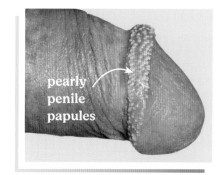

pearly penile papules

Painful Penis Problems (See Your Doctor)

When your penis is in pain, have no shame—get to a doctor ASAP. It might be nothing, but it could be something that will only get worse over time, like a sexually transmitted infection (see page 185 for more).

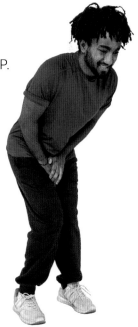

✦ **Pain when retracting foreskin.** Usually, an uncircumcised person should be able to easily retract (pull back) their foreskin behind the head of their penis by the time they've started puberty, and some by the age of five. When erect ("hard"), the foreskin naturally retracts, but sometimes retraction is painful and/or impossible, and this is called phimosis. This condition is often diagnosed in young children; however, some STIs can cause it, as can forcibly pulling the foreskin back, which leads to scarring. See your doctor to rule out larger problems where phimosis is a symptom and to find options and exercises to help you regain the ability to retract your foreskin.

+ **Foreskin remains retracted.** Sometimes an uncircumcised person's foreskin stays retracted and refuses to go back to covering the head of the penis, even when flaccid (soft). This is called paraphimosis. Because the foreskin remains retracted, it can affect blood flow to the head of the penis, causing pain and swelling. It can sometimes go away on its own, but medical intervention might be needed, and the sooner you seek help, the faster you can heal. When in doubt, have it checked out!

+ **Head of penis hurts.** Sometimes the glans or foreskin can become inflamed and feel painful and itchy, occasionally even oozing discharge from developed sores. This is called balanitis (or balanoposthitis in uncircumcised people) and can be caused by an STI (see page 185), an allergic reaction, a buildup of bacteria and bodily fluids from not washing properly (page 10), or by a fungal infection (page 42). See your doctor to get a diagnosis and the proper medication to heal.

+ **Penis skin stuck to shaft.** Occasionally, a person's glans (head) becomes adhered (glued) to the shaft (long part) of the penis, whether circumcised or uncircumcised. This is called a penile adhesion, and a common symptom is tugging or pain felt during an erection, which can make masturbation or intercourse difficult. Some penile adhesions repair themselves, but others require medical intervention. Many people unnecessarily suffer uncomfortable erections due to penile adhesions for years because of fear or shame, but doctors see penile adhesions all the time, so what are you waiting for?

Zipper Accidents (Ouch!)

Have you ever pulled up your zip and gotten your penis nipped? If so, you know this can be extremely painful. But sometimes, a quick zip turns into a complete ordeal, as the penis can accidentally get caught up in the zipper. OUCH! If this happens to you, do NOT unzip and seek medical attention ASAP. Zipper teeth can cause a lot of damage to the penis, and trying to do DIY removal might worsen your problem. See your doctor immediately, as not only will you need help getting your penis out of the zipper, but also your penis may need professional repair. Fortunately, the doctor can likely provide an anesthetic, so you won't have to feel the process of removal and repair. Zipper accidents are the most common cause of penile injuries—so zip with care (or wear underwear)!

> People with penises can get urinary tract infections, too! If it hurts to pee, see page 108 for more on urinary tract infections (UTIs).

Unhealthy Penile Discharge

Discharge is any liquid that comes from your urethra that isn't urine. While people born with vaginas have a lot of reasons to produce many kinds of healthy discharge (see page 157), the urethral opening of people with penises should not normally produce anything that isn't urine, smegma (page 126), pre-ejaculate, or ejaculate (page 140). If this happens to you, see your doctor, as there is likely inflammation or an infection (such as a urinary tract infection, but possibly a sexually transmitted one like the gonorrhea discharge pictured on the right) that requires a proper diagnosis.

gonorrhea

When there's a fungal infection around the genitalia but not on it, it's referred to as jock itch—see page 42 for more.

Scrotums and Testicles

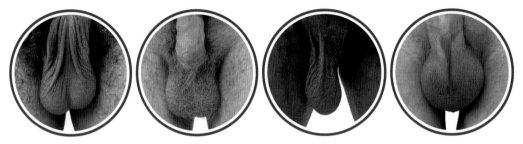

Under the penis is a baggy sack of skin called the scrotum. The scrotum contains the testicles, which are primary reproductive organs that produce hormones and sperm (see page 164 for more on hormones). The scrotum is also an erogenous zone, meaning it feels really good to touch.

Before birth, testicles develop inside the body of people born with penises, and they usually make their way down into the scrotum at some point before birth. However, sometimes a person is born with an undescended testicle, which is when one or both testicles remain inside the body after birth. This is usually caught and either monitored or addressed through surgery as an infant, but if you have a scrotum and notice that it feels like it's missing a testicle inside, see your doctor so they can monitor and discuss possible treatment options, as people with undescended testicles are at higher risk of developing testicular cancer, whether or not it's corrected.

Testicles don't always like to stay in their place! Sometimes testicles are retractile, which means they can retreat back into the body. This can be normal, especially if they're always able to eventually make their way back down to the scrotum. Fear, cold temperatures, and even touch can cause testicles to unexpectedly travel. Still, if one or both of your testicles tend to disappear, see your doctor, who can keep tabs over time to make sure everything is okay.

Testicular Injury

Whether a baseball lands between your legs or someone thinks it's funny to kick you in the testicles (it's not), if you have testicular pain for more than a couple of hours, see your doctor, as injury to this area should be taken seriously.

Your doctor can make sure it's not something more problematic like testicular torsion, which can happen when the cord that supplies blood to the testicles gets twisted, causing one or both testicles to swell and become extremely painful. Aside from injury, testicle growth during puberty can cause testicular torsion, too—that's why most people who deal with testicular torsion are under eighteen years old.

To prevent testicular injury during sports, wear an athletic cup, which is a hard shell to protect the penis and testicles. And if you hang out with people who think it's funny to punch or kick people "in the balls," make them stop! Repeated injury to the penis and testicles is not only painful but can cause permanent testicular damage.

How to Perform a Testicular Self-Exam

Testicular cancer is the most common cancer diagnosed in people born with penises between the ages of fifteen and forty, and it's on the rise. Similar to being "breast and chest aware" (see page 86), it's important to know what your scrotum and testicles usually look and feel like so you can quickly seek help if something seems off.

Fortunately, giving yourself a testicular self-exam is quick and easy!

Try to examine yourself once a month when you're relaxed and in a private place, ideally in the shower. (The shower's warm steam can also make your scrotum easier to check.) If you prefer to check outside the shower, sometimes it's helpful to place one foot on a chair or the toilet lid to gain better access to the area.

First, gently move your penis aside and give your scrotum a visual inspection—grab a mirror if you need to, and don't forget the underside. There should be two testicles in the scrotal sac—if not, see page 134 for information on undescended testicles. Often, one testicle is larger or hangs lower in the scrotum—this is totally normal. In fact, often the right one is larger and the left one hangs lower. However, if you're worried about the size and shape of your scrotum and testicles, see your doctor.

Next, use your fingers to examine how each testicle feels physically. Choose one to start and stabilize your testicle by gently pinching your thumb and pointer finger at the top of your scrotum, with your other fingers placed underneath.

While still holding the top of the scrotum, use the fingers and thumb from your other hand to feel the testicle—which should be round, smooth, and firm (but not rock hard). Check for any lumps or bumps along the testicle's front, back, and sides. You should feel a spermatic cord running behind and above each testicle, connecting it to the body. The first time you examine yourself you may be surprised to feel a soft structure near the top of the back of each testicle that is sensitive to touch—that's the epididymis, which stores sperm from the testicles. Remember where it is so you won't mistake it for a new lump in the future.

Finally, gently roll the testicle with your fingers for a few seconds as a final lump check.

Repeat the process with the other testicle.

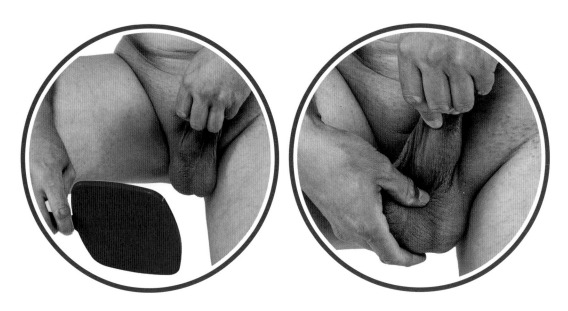

Once you have a baseline for how things normally look and feel, write down any new developments, and see your doctor if you:

- ✦ Feel testicular aches, tenderness, or pains

- ✦ Notice changes in the size or color of your scrotum or testicles

- ✦ Find new bumps, lumps, or swelling. If you see new bumps or lumps and you're sexually active, it could be an STI (see page 127 for more on genital bumps)

There are many reasons you might have testicular pain or lumps that aren't cancerous but still could benefit from a doctor's examination—a hernia, cyst, or infection being some common issues. Sometimes your testicular veins can get larger and cause lumpiness, too—this is called a varicocele and often is described as feeling like a bag of worms in the scrotum. Any sudden onset of testicular pain or swelling is important to have checked out ASAP to make sure there is not a blood-flow issue to your testicle called a testicular torsion (see page 135).

Even if it is testicular cancer, it is extremely curable (95 to 99 percent) when caught and treated early. So don't delay—check yourself today!

> If you're a person with limited mobility, giving yourself a thorough testicular exam may be difficult or impossible, but these exams are still an important part of your preventative care. Talk to your doctor about alternate strategies so that you can best care for your body.

From Flaccid to Erect

The penis has two states: flaccid (soft) and erect (hard). A soft penis can appear very different from a hard one—often, it doesn't even look like the same penis!

An erection happens when blood from other parts of the body rushes into the shaft and glans, where muscles tighten up to trap the blood. The trapped blood expands the penis, making it harder, longer, straighter, and wider (erect).

Have you ever heard penises referred to as "show-ers" vs. "grow-ers?" That's because sometimes a penis doesn't get much larger when it's erect (a show-er); but other times, it can tremendously increase in size (a grow-er).

Types of Erections

Erections can be expected, meaning the trigger is known, or they can be spontaneous (unexpected), meaning the penis becomes erect "on its own," whether or not an erection is welcome.

Spontaneous erections are common, especially in the first few years of puberty. But just because they're common doesn't mean they aren't frustrating to deal with, especially when erections happen at the most inopportune times (like while giving a speech in front of the entire class).

Erections occur for a variety of reasons—they even happen in the womb! Three main causes are:

+ **Physical touch.** If you have a penis, you probably already know that pleasurable touch (from yourself or others) can cause an erection. But many types of touch can spark a spontaneous erection—a cool breeze, vibrations from a massage chair, friction from clothing, etc. Touching other body parts, especially erogenous (pleasurable) zones like the nipple or mouth, can also cause an erection.

+ **Thoughts and emotions.** Thinking about someone you're attracted to can cause sexual arousal, which can lead to an erection. Nonsexual thoughts can cause surprise, spontaneous erections—like remembering something exciting that happened to you. Feeling nervous or embarrassed can cause a sudden erection, too, so if your stress about getting an erection causes you to get an erection, you're not psychic; you're just normal!

+ **Sleeping.** Quite a few spontaneous erections can happen during sleep— between three to six each night. When you wake up and your penis is saluting you, that's its final spontaneous erection of the night. These types of erections may or may not be from sexual dreams.

Other reasons erections can happen include physical exercise and having to urinate.

There's no right number of erections to have each day, and it's not possible to have "too many" or "too few." However, if you have an erection that is painful or will not go away (and you've tried everything in the next section to bring it down), see your doctor. Erections should feel good, not bad! More on this on page 142.

Some scientists think that morning erections are the body's reaction to having a full bladder as a way to prevent bed-wetting. There's nothing conclusive, but perhaps that's why people with penises usually have to wait until a morning erection goes down before they can pee.

Back to Flaccid

A penis stays erect until the muscles relax, allowing the blood to escape. Once the blood has left the penis, it returns to its usual flaccid state. This can take anywhere from a minute or two to half an hour.

Two ways to help an erect penis "deflate" are:

+ **Distract yourself from it.** When an erection is ignored long enough, the muscles eventually relax, draining the trapped blood and softening the penis. Finding something to distract your mind can speed things up, such as watching television or playing a game on your phone.

+ **Focus on it until orgasm.** You can also deflate an erection by focusing on it until pleasurable feelings build up to an exciting peak, called an orgasm. Orgasming, also known as "coming" or "climaxing," can be brought on in a variety of ways, including masturbating (touching yourself for sexual pleasure), during sleep (see page 141 for info on nocturnal emissions), and sexual activity (more on safe sex on page 174).

Ejaculation (Orgasm)

Usually, when people born with penises and testicles orgasm, a thick, whitish fluid called semen is "ejected" out of the tip of the penis through the urethra. This process is called ejaculation, which is why semen is also formally known as ejaculate. Semen contains sperm, which, when combined with eggs from people born with ovaries, can create a baby (more on reproduction on page 171).

While it can seem like a lot of liquid when it shoots out, most ejaculations are less than 1 teaspoon of fluid.

Right after an erect penis ejaculates, the muscles immediately relax and the trapped blood that helped create the erection can then escape, bringing the penis back to its flaccid state.

> It's possible to ejaculate without orgasm, and it's possible to orgasm with little or no ejaculated semen. However you ejaculate, the experience is meant to always feel good; see your doctor if ejaculation hurts or is uncomfortable.

Pre-come Can Put the Pre- in Pregnancy (and the Sigh in STI)

Don't believe the lies—pre-come absolutely can transmit disease and cause pregnancy! Pre-ejaculate, also known as pre-come, is a clear, thin fluid that leaks out of the tip of an erect penis before ejaculation. While pre-come doesn't contain sperm itself, it can become contaminated with sperm in the urethra. It can also transmit STIs, so it is important to always use protection before starting any genitalia-to-genitalia contact that involves a penis (see page 178 for types of protection available to prevent STIs and pregnancy).

> See page 146 for more information on orgasms for people born with vaginas!

Wet Dreams (Nocturnal Emissions)

Waking up from a deep sleep with semen-soaked bedsheets can come as a shock, especially the first time it happens (which may be a person's first experience with ejaculation). Commonly known as "wet dreams" and also as "nocturnal emissions" (even though they can happen during a daytime nap, too), spontaneous erections that end in orgasm while sleeping are common, normal, and healthy.

> People without testicles and people born with vaginas have "wet dreams," too! Theirs just aren't usually as "wet" due to the fact that they don't have the organs to produce semen (but know that a moist vagina is super healthy; see page 157 for more).

Broken Penis

While penises don't have bones, when erect (hard), they can be fractured (broken) if harshly bent or twisted. Sexual intercourse is the number one cause of penile fractures, but it can also happen during other sexual activities, like masturbation.

Signs of a fractured penis include:

+ A cracking or popping sound when the injury happens

+ Pain, bruising, or swelling on the penis after the injury

+ Blood in urine or on the penis

See your doctor (or go to the emergency room if it's extremely painful, which it probably will be) as soon as possible if you notice any of these symptoms—don't delay because of embarrassment or shame! While penile fractures are uncommon, when they happen, they can be severe enough to require surgery.

Painful Erections

Erections should NOT be painful! Sometimes, erections can feel painful because of penile adhesions (see page 132 for more). If a painful erection lasts longer than four hours and won't go away, that is called priapism. Erections from priapism usually aren't sexual and are often a symptom of another illness (like sickle cell anemia). If this happens to you, see your doctor *immediately,* as this can cause permanent damage to your penis if not medically treated.

Erectile Dysfunction

At certain times in a person's life, it can become harder to get hard. It tends to be easier for people in their teens and early twenties to become erect because there's more of the hormone testosterone surging through the body, but stress, illness, weight changes, penile fractures (see page 141), certain medications, and recreational drugs are some of the issues that can cause difficulty achieving and keeping an erection. This is also known as erectile dysfunction or impotence. If this happens to you, it's normal and can usually be resolved. See your doctor so they can check you for any medical issues for which impotence is a symptom, like diabetes and depression.

Blue Balls (and Blue Vulva)

Sometimes testicles hurt because an erect penis close to orgasm stops being stimulated, which can cause a slight ache until the erection eventually goes down. Even though it has a medical name, epididymal hypertension, "blue balls" is NOT a serious condition that can damage the body in any way, contrary to popular myths. When it happens to people with vaginas, it's called "blue vulva," or some say "blue bean," due to the shape of the clitoral glans (keep reading for more on vulvas and clitorises).

While there is discomfort, there is no danger, so if "blue balls" or "blue vulva" happens to you, there is NO medical reason to force orgasm, and you should NEVER try to force an orgasm with an uninterested person out of fear of "feeling blue." (Nor should any sexual contact be forced upon you ever; see page 185 for information on sexual assault).

So whether you were interrupted while masturbating or your sexual partner no longer wants to participate, just take a deep breath, focus on something else, and your genitalia will eventually return to its unstimulated state.

Vulvas

What many people call the vagina is actually the vulva. The vulva isn't just one body organ but a collection of external (visible) genitalia that includes:

+ **The mons pubis.** The mound of skin and pubic hair that cushions the pelvic bone, where most of the pubic hair grows. All people have a mons, and sometimes people are worried that theirs is too puffy or prominent, but it's designed that way on purpose! Know that all mons are fabulous and there's nothing weird or bad about your body the way it is.

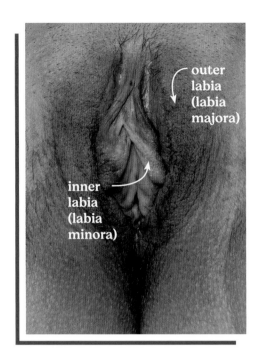

✦ **The outer labia (*labia majora*) and inner labia (*labia minora*).** Sensitive folds of skin that act like security doors to the vaginal opening, protecting it from harm. They're also erogenous zones, meaning they feel really good to touch. The outer labia are covered in pubic hair (if not removed). Inside the outer labia are the inner labia, which can grow hair, too, but generally less hair than the outer labia. Labial folds vary tremendously in length, appearance, and even symmetry—one study found that the left inner labia is often slightly longer than the right.

Sometimes a fluid-filled growth called a Bartholin's cyst can form when glands become blocked on the labia of people born with vaginas. Bartholin's cysts generally are only found on one side of the vulva, near the vaginal opening. Often, these lumps are small and painless, but finding one can still be scary, especially if you're sexually active, as they can look and feel a lot like an STI. They sometimes go away on their own, but see your doctor if your labia lump stays for more than a couple of days or if it becomes uncomfortable or painful in any way, as you may have an infection. (See page 127 for info on other bumps that might appear elsewhere on your vulva.)

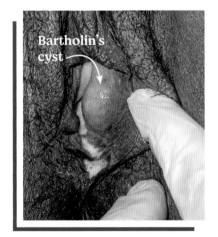

- **The clitoral glans.** The bean-like tip of the clitoris visible at the top of the vulva, just above the urethral opening. It is one of the body's most powerful erogenous zones, meaning it's a supersensitive and very pleasurable place to touch. Clitoral stimulation is one of the ways people can reach orgasm (see page 146 for more).

- **The clitoral hood.** This skin fold covers the tip of the clitoral glans. When excited by sexual touch or thoughts, the clitoral hood retracts as the clitoris swells with blood and becomes larger and even more sensitive, similar to an erect penis.

- **The urethral opening.** Just below the clitoral glans is the opening to the urethra, which is the tube through which urine exits the body.

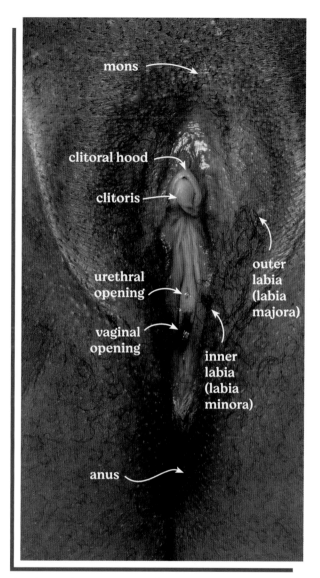

mons

clitoral hood

clitoris

urethral opening

vaginal opening

anus

outer labia (labia majora)

inner labia (labia minora)

(Pardon the blood; this person's period made a surprise appearance during our photo shoot!)

- **The vaginal opening.** Underneath the urethral opening is the opening to the vagina. (Keep reading for more on vaginas.)

The entire clitoris is way bigger than the part you can see! Inside the body the clitoris has multiple portions, and the total size can be about the same as the external part of the penis. That shouldn't be surprising, considering that penises and clitorises both develop in the womb from the same genital tissue.

Orgasm

Orgasm is the height of pleasure from sexual thoughts or touches. Admittedly, that's a pretty boring description for something that can feel so wonderful! People with vaginas can achieve orgasm in a variety of ways—masturbation, which is touching oneself for the purpose of pleasure; sexual activity; or even just sexual thoughts, both conscious and subconscious (see page 141 for information on "wet dreams").

Stimulating the clitoris can play a huge role in orgasm, as can touch in other erogenous zones, such as the labia, vagina, nipples, perineum, mouth, and other sensitive body parts.

While some fluid can be released during orgasm, people with vaginas generally don't ejaculate like those born with the organs that make semen. Some people born with vaginas release a large amount of fluid after orgasm, and while scientists have yet to figure out what it is, studies have determined that it isn't urine.

See page 140 for more information on orgasm for people born with penises!

Vaginas

You can't see your vagina, but it's there—and extremely important. The vagina is a tunnel-shaped organ that connects the vulva to the rest of the internal genitalia, including reproductive organs like the uterus and fallopian tubes. Like vulvas, all vaginas are a little different—they can be wide, narrow, long, short . . . there's no one "right" vaginal shape. One thing all vaginas have in common, however, is that vaginal tissue is very stretchy. The amount a vagina can stretch (and contract) at any given time depends on various factors, like sexual arousal and hormone levels. Menstrual blood (see page 148) flows from the uterus and exits the body out of the vagina, as can babies, which is why another name for the vagina is the "birth canal."

Vaginal and/or Vulvar Pain (See Your Doctor)

Don't be ashamed—see your doctor immediately if you're dealing with vaginal or vulvar pain!

It's not uncommon for people, especially young adults, to ignore this kind of pain for weeks, or even months, hoping it will go away. When this happens, everyday activities like exercising, using internal menstrual products, and even wearing underwear can become difficult and uncomfortable. Because it can be tough to talk about genitalia, many think that this type of pain and suffering is acceptable, but it's not! There are many reasons a vulva or vagina can be painful, including:

+ **Vaginal or vulvar tears.** It's not uncommon to injure your delicate vaginal or vulvar skin, especially after any kind of penetration, whether that's from a tampon, a finger, a penis, or something else. Talk to your doctor, who has probably seen hundreds of issues similar to yours, to make sure you're healing properly and to rule out infection.

+ **Bartholin's cysts.** Cysts can be very painful and sometimes need to be professionally popped. See page 144 for more.

+ **Infections.** Sexually transmitted infections (see page 185) and other infections, like yeast (page 158) can cause pain. See your doctor to get a diagnosis and treatment to manage or clear the infection.

✦ **Medical conditions.** Certain painful conditions like vulvodynia, vaginismus, or vaginitis can make any type of vaginal insertion challenging or impossible. These issues can last for months and sometimes come about after an infection clears, but often show up for no reason at all. If you're stuck with lingering pain and your doctor can't figure out why, mention these possible conditions to your doctor, as there are treatment options available, including physical therapy.

It's almost never possible to properly diagnose or treat yourself, and it's important to never be shy about seeking help for any type of pain, especially "down there." Again, see your doctor to get help and hopefully rule out (or treat) something serious.

> It's very common for people to not feel well right before or during their period, as menstruation often comes with vaginal or vulvar pain, nausea, headaches, back pains, bloating (see page 112), and cramping (page 152).

Menstruation (Your Period)

Menstruation ("having a period") is a huge part of life for most people born with a uterus and a vagina. It's natural, normal, healthy . . . and messy.

Every month or so, starting after puberty begins, a menstruating body starts a new cycle as it prepares for the possibility of reproduction (see page 171 for more). Hormones trigger a process called ovulation, when one of the body's two ovaries releases an egg. That egg travels through one of the fallopian tubes to the uterus, where it then hangs out in a thick layer of blood and tissue called the uterine lining.

If semen enters the vagina, sperm can travel to the egg and fertilize it. If this happens, when the fertilized egg makes its way to the uterus, the uterine lining nourishes it as it develops into an embryo. If the egg is not fertilized, the uterine lining absorbs it after a few days. Then muscles in the uterus contract to push the lining out of the body through the vaginal canal.

The expelled lining is commonly called menstrual blood, or your period. It can range in color and texture from fresh, thin, bright-red blood to thicker, darker-colored tissue and blood. An average period might look like a whole lot, but the uterus usually only releases about 5 tablespoons of blood (though an extremely heavy period can produce over ten times that amount).

Sometimes menstrual blood contains clots, which are chunks of blood that have coagulated (stuck together). A few quarter-sized or smaller clots a day during menstruation are normal.

It usually takes three to seven days for the uterus to completely empty out. When this happens, menstrual bleeding stops and the cycle begins again: the uterus regrows a new lining, awaits a new egg, and then either pregnancy or menstruation occurs.

Even though menstrual cycles are usually referred to as happening "once a month," they rarely run like clockwork. In some months, menstrual blood flow may be heavy and last for a week, while in other months, there might only be brown mucus for a couple of days. These fluctuations are normal.

See page 171 for more details on eggs, semen, sperm, embryos, and reproduction!

Heavy Periods

It's difficult to judge exactly how heavy menstrual flow is when it's happening—no one's standing with a measuring cup between their legs for days, right?

A simple way to estimate if flow is heavier than expected for an average period is to take note of how often period products need to be changed.

Two signs of a heavier-than-normal period are:

+ Needing to change menstrual products every single hour for six hours in a row

+ Having a period that lasts for more than seven days

If you notice one or both of these symptoms, see your doctor and tell them the specifics about your menstrual flow. If the bleeding is affecting your ability to live your normal life when you menstruate, you may be dealing with menorrhagia, which is the medical term for heavy menstrual bleeding. Menorrhagia is a symptom of many period-related issues, including the ones discussed on page 153.

> Not every person born with a vagina menstruates, but if you don't, it's important to figure out why. See your doctor if menstruation hasn't begun by age fifteen. They can examine you and screen for various causes of a delayed or missing period, such as an intersex variation. In fact, some people find out they are intersex because they don't ever get a period, with lack of menstruation being the only external sign. See page 167–68 for more on intersex variations.

Missing Periods

Every person who menstruates misses a period or two at some point in their lives. Maybe an egg wasn't produced, or there may just not be enough uterine lining to shed. The first few years of menstruating (shortly after puberty begins) are often irregular, but there are many reasons anyone could miss a period, including:

+ Exercising more or eating less

+ Losing or gaining weight suddenly

+ Getting sick

- ✦ Having lots of stress (mental or physical)

- ✦ Having certain medical conditions (keep reading for more)

- ✦ Traveling through different time zones

- ✦ Taking a new medication

Of course, missing a period is also a sign of pregnancy, which can be a big worry for people who are sexually active. In this situation, it's important to take a pregnancy test as soon as possible and every few days after until either a period or a positive test shows up. See page 174 for more on sexual health.

> Between puberty and menopause, a total of 2,280 days, or over six years of life, can be spent bleeding during more than 450 menstrual periods unless menstruation is medically suppressed due to illness, pregnancy, or hormonal birth control (see page 182 for more).

If pregnancy tests are negative (or if you haven't been sexually active) and three or more menstrual cycles are skipped, it may be an issue called secondary amenorrhea, which is the lack of a period in a person who has previously been menstruating. While secondary amenorrhea isn't life-threatening, it is usually a symptom of a more serious problem, such as low body weight or a hormonal imbalance like endometriosis (see page 153) or polycystic ovary syndrome (PCOS; see page 153). A doctor can run tests to find out exactly why menstruation stopped and how to get it back on track.

> People who use hormonal birth control may notice that their period is very light or even stops. This is because hormonal birth control prevents an ovary from releasing an egg (a process called ovulation, which is discussed on page 148). Without ovulation, very little blood and tissue builds up in the uterine lining, causing a light period (or none at all). For more on types of birth control, see page 181.

Period Tracking

Tracking menstrual cycles is very helpful in knowing with certainty if a period has been missed, came early, or lasts too long. After a few months of tracking, patterns might start to appear—when cramps and other pain peak, what moods and emotions to expect, and when to start wearing menstrual products to avoid period stains.

While using a product specifically made for period tracking, like a notebook or phone app, is probably easier, especially for those with irregular menstrual cycles, the body already has a built-in tracking system: vaginal discharge. Learning how to frequently check vaginal discharge to track period patterns (using the information about types of discharge on page 157) can be interesting, rewarding, and eventually instant—once a person knows what type of discharge their body tends to produce right before a period, they won't even need to wait for the phone app's warning!

> A normal menstrual cycle is roughly between three and six weeks (twenty-one and forty-five days) for teenagers. See your doctor if you get your period more often or less frequently than that on a regular basis.

Cramps

Most people who menstruate experience cramps. Formally known as dysmenorrhea, which means "painful monthly bleeding" in Greek, cramps usually start right before a period, when hormones cause muscles in the uterus to contract in order to push out the uterine lining (menstrual blood). Aside from abdominal bloating and aches and pains, dysmenorrhea can also include headaches, nausea and vomiting, exhaustion, and even changes in poop, like constipation or diarrhea.

Cramps tend to be the most painful on the heaviest day of blood flow, and they dull as the period ends. If cramps are, well, *cramping* your style, there are a few things you can try to help manage this painful part of your period, including:

- **Over-the-counter pain-relieving pills.** These help to dull the pain, especially if taken as soon as the first aches are felt. Always read and follow the instructions on the bottle or box about proper dosage for your body weight and age.

- **Heat on your abdomen**. A hot water bottle, heating pad, or warm bath or shower can reduce pain by relaxing the uterine muscles (and you).

- **Light exercise or yoga.** Gentle movements can help relax the contracting muscles, too. Exercise also releases endorphins, which are hormones your body produces that have the ability to help the body feel better.

> If you're cramping and curious, many people find some relief by masturbating to orgasm, which not only feels great but also can relieve menstrual cramps. No one is exactly sure why, but one reason might be that masturbating to orgasm can release stress-reducing hormones that act as natural pain killers!

Severe Cramps (and Possible Reasons Why)

Unfortunately, for some people—including a lot of teen menstruators—cramps are so intense that menstrual periods disrupt their lives, causing them to miss school or work at least once every menstrual cycle. If you find yourself plagued by severe period cramps, see your doctor, who can check for more serious problems that have cramping as a side effect, including:

- **Fibroids.** Up to 70 percent of menstruating people will develop fibroids, which are growths that can form outside or inside of the uterus and can cause extreme cramping.

- **Polycystic ovary syndrome (PCOS).** Up to 12 percent of people who menstruate are diagnosed with PCOS, which is a hormone imbalance that can cause painful cramping, even when not menstruating. PCOS can also cause acne (see page 19), excessive hair growth (page 56), hyperpigmentation (page 38), weight gain, and fertility issues.

✦ **Endometriosis.** More than 11 percent of people who menstruate suffer from this extremely painful condition, which is when excess uterine tissue grows outside of the uterus.

✦ **Cysts.** About 10 percent of people who menstruate experience ovarian cysts, which are sacs filled with fluid that develop on one or both ovaries and can cause painful cramps.

See your doctor, as only a medical professional can truly diagnose any of these conditions and prescribe medication, such as hormonal birth control, to help.

> Scientists are starting to see a relationship between what a person eats and menstrual cramps. People who eat more sugar and drink more coffee may be prone to heavier and more painful cramping.

PMS and PMDD

The week or so before menstrual blood starts to flow, hormone fluctuations can cause up to 90 percent of menstruators to experience a variety of emotional shifts and physical changes known as premenstrual syndrome (PMS for short). Sometimes people like to joke about whether or not someone's "PMSing," but the symptoms can feel like no laughing matter.

Common emotional symptoms include changes in mood and appetite, feelings of anxiety and depression, and heightened emotions. PMS can also be paired with cramping and other physical symptoms, like headaches, bloating, breast tenderness, and tiredness.

Sometimes PMS symptoms are more severe, like near-constant crying or not being able to sleep or concentrate. When PMS affects the quality of a person's life in these or other ways, it's called premenstrual dysphoric disorder (PMDD), which happens to up to 8 percent of people who menstruate.

Different treatments work for different people. Most PMS-minimizing suggestions are similar to those for cramping, and include doctor-prescribed and over-the-counter medicine, exercise for natural pain-killing endorphins, and rest.

See your doctor if PMS or PMDD symptoms are interfering with your life. They can help rule out more serious illnesses with similar symptoms as well as possibly prescribe medication that might help.

> Menstrual cycles tend to continue regularly for over forty years until menopause, which is when hormones stop triggering ovulation, so no eggs are released into the uterus. With no eggs to potentially fertilize, the body stops producing uterine lining, ending the menstrual cycle. Menopause generally happens between the ages of forty-five and fifty-five.

Types of Menstrual Products

There are two types of menstrual products:

- **External menstrual products.** These products catch menstrual blood as it exits the vaginal opening.

- **Internal menstrual products.** These products are inserted into the vagina to collect menstrual blood internally.

All types of menstrual products must be changed often to prevent odor, irritation, leaks, and—in the case of internal menstrual products—toxic shock syndrome (TSS; see page 157).

External menstrual products include:

◆ **Disposable pads.** The most common period product in the world is the pad. Also known as a sanitary napkin, it's a rectangular-shaped pad (of various lengths and thicknesses) made of absorbent materials with adhesive on the back to temporarily stick to underwear. It absorbs menstrual fluid and must be changed and discarded multiple times each day. Pads come in many different absorption levels, from extremely thin panty liners meant for very light period days or heavy vaginal discharge days (see page 157) to larger, extremely absorbent overnight options.

◆ **Reusable pads.** These function in the same way as disposable pads, except they are designed to be washed, dried, and reused multiple times. They're made of sturdier fabrics like cotton, fleece, or wool, have snaps or buttons instead of adhesive, and often have a waterproof lining sewn in.

◆ **Period underwear.** This is like regular underwear, but with extra padding in the crotch area to directly absorb menstrual blood; no other product is needed. Often there is a waterproof lining sewn in. Different absorbency levels are available—period underwear designed to hold more blood tends to be bulkier and less flexible than pairs for spotting or light flow. Period underwear is reusable. Most people need at least five pairs to get through their cycle because wearing a single pair longer than twelve hours isn't recommended due to odor and leaks.

Internal menstrual products include:

◆ **Tampons.** The most popular internal menstrual product is a tube of absorbent material called a tampon. It's usually (and preferably) cotton or a mix of cotton and other synthetic fibers. Tampons should be changed every four to eight hours, and more often on heavy flow days. Some people find it easier to time their tampon changes to whenever they have to pee.

✦ **Cups and discs.** Menstrual cups are flexible containers that can fold for vaginal insertion, then pop back into a cup shape once inside the vagina. Menstrual cups are usually reusable after washing and are designed to be changed less frequently than tampons—sometimes only a couple of times a day, depending upon flow. Menstrual discs work like cups, but are larger and thus need to be changed even less frequently. Their Frisbee-esque shape can take some getting used to when it comes to mess-free removal, but people who get the hang of discs say that the extra capacity and barely there feel are true benefits over other product options. There are both reusable and disposable discs available for purchase.

Toxic Shock Syndrome

If a tampon, cup, or disc is left in the vaginal canal for too long, bacteria can grow and make the menstruating person sick with a very dangerous condition called toxic shock syndrome (TSS). TSS is easy to prevent by simply changing internal menstrual products (tampon, cup, or disc) according to the manufacturer's instructions, which is usually every four to eight hours, depending upon flow heaviness. The longer you wait, the more time bacteria have to begin their infectious growth. Alternating between internal and external menstrual products and using the proper absorbency for your flow (so you have to change it out more often) can help prevent infections, too. But don't immediately panic if you forget to change your tampon. TSS used to be more common when tampons had higher absorbencies (meaning they could hold more menstrual blood). The lower absorbency of modern tampons makes it difficult to absorb enough blood to cause TSS . . . but not impossible. See your doctor ASAP if you start having flu-like symptoms such as feeling faint or confused, vomiting, diarrhea, or a high fever.

Vaginal Discharge

A well-functioning vagina is supposed to be moist, but the type and quantity of discharge that vaginas produce change from day to day. On heavy discharge days it can help to wear a menstrual product, such as period underwear or a pad/panty liner to avoid discomfort from walking around in wet underwear. Don't be surprised if, like nose boogers, vaginal discharge becomes crusty when it dries. That's totally normal (especially if it's smegma; see page 126 for more).

Different colors, smells, and textures indicate various phases of the menstrual cycle (see page 148 for more on menstruation) and can also signify whether something's not quite right.

Any of the following symptoms might be a sign of something being awry:

+ Unusually colored discharge

+ Unexpected or stinky smells and/or textures

+ More than usual discharge

+ Pain, burning, or itchiness

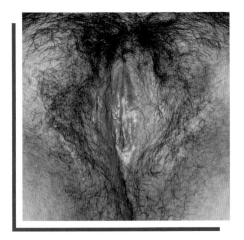

The day of our shoot was a heavy discharge day for this person, who has a healthy and moist vagina. Your nose produces mucus to stay healthy, and similarly, vaginas produce discharge—up to a teaspoon a day—in order to protect against infections and flush out old cells.

If vaginal discharge matches any of these descriptions, there are a few possibile causes, including:

+ **Forgotten internal period product.** Old tampons or a menstrual cup left too long in the vagina can cause stinky, colored discharge.

+ **Yeast infection.** Excess yeast in the vagina can cause an itchy infection that is usually odorless but comes with a white, clumpy discharge. Most people with vaginas get at least one yeast infection in their lives, and many suffer from frequent infections (see page 43 for prevention info). Wiping front-to-back and keeping your body clean and dry can help with prevention, but some people are just prone to getting them. Over-the-counter medicine or doctor-prescribed treatments usually clear the yeast infection in a week.

+ **Bacterial vaginosis (BV).** If vaginal discharge has a funky odor, chances are this super common infection is the cause, especially if the discharge is milky. Up to one-third of those born with vaginas get BV at some point, but the reasons why are unknown. If BV is left untreated too long, the infection can spread to the rest of the reproductive organs, so it's important to see your doctor and get checked out. Fortunately, a simple prescription antibiotic can clear BV in no time.

+ **Urinary tract infection (UTI).** Discharge is sometimes a sign of a UTI, along with pain while urinating, stinky and/or cloudy urine, and a frequent need to urinate. More on UTIs on page 108.

+ **Sexually transmitted infections (STIs).** Some STIs are associated with greenish-yellow, and sometimes smelly, discharge. There's no way you can know if the discharge is because of chlamydia, trichomoniasis, or another issue, so it's very important to see your doctor so they can identify the cause of the discharge. See page 185 for more on STIs.

A gynecologist is a type of doctor that helps people with vaginas care for their reproductive system. See page 192 for more on types of doctors.

How to Learn Vaginal Discharge Patterns

If you have a vagina and want to learn your discharge pattern (perhaps to predict your period, as discussed on page 151), it's easy to do a quick finger check each morning.

First, wash your hands and gently insert your pointer finger into your vagina and wiggle it around. You might be surprised by how soft and wet it is—that's exactly how it's supposed to be. When you're ready, pull out your finger and press it into your thumb. Then slowly separate the two digits, noting what the discharge does and comparing it to the following guide:

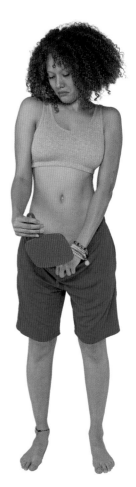

+ **When ovulating,** a sticky, clear liquid usually means that an egg is ready to be fertilized.

+ **During menstruation,** vaginas shed a bloody, often clot-filled discharge containing the unfertilized egg and other uterine tissues.

+ **Right after menstruation,** a brown, gummy discharge is normal (that's just old blood leaving the system).

+ **At other times,** generally speaking, discharge is all right if it's clear, yellowish, or white. But if it's stinky or itchy? Something's fishy, so see your doctor.

Early lunar (moon-based) calendars often had thirteen months because they were based on the phases of the moon, which also happens to be the average length of menstrual cycles, with each month having twenty-eight days.

To Douche or Not to Douche?

The answer is almost always no! (See sidebar for an exception.) While it's very important for people born with vaginas to wash their vulvas (external genitalia) every day, cleaning inside the vaginal canal is unnecessary and might even cause harm. Vaginal douching—the act of squirting water or special cleansers into the vagina—is often believed to help keep a vagina "fresh," but that's not true. The body automatically produces vaginal discharge that is perfectly capable of thoroughly cleaning the vaginal canal all by itself. Douching does not prevent STIs, and people born with vaginas who douche are actually more likely to suffer from potentially stinky and uncomfortable vaginal infections as well as abnormal discharge.

So instead of buying prepackaged douches that claim to improve vaginal odor and health, try keeping clean with the tips on page 13 instead. And if something seems off, instead of douching, see your doctor to find out if you simply have a stinky infection that the right medicine can clear up.

> Under the supervision of their healthcare team, trans women and intersex people who have had a vagina surgically created usually need to douche their vagina to keep it clean.

sex, gender & sexual health

IT'S A GIRL!   IT'S A BABY!   IT'S A BOY!

We tend to think of the word "sex" in terms of the physical activity. But sex can also mean one of the categories that people are assigned to at birth based on their external genitalia.

Immediately after a baby is born, someone looks between their legs to assign a sex on the baby's birth certificate. "It's a boy!" is declared for people born with penises, who are then assigned male at birth (AMAB for short). "It's a girl!" is for people born with vulvas, who are assigned female at birth (AFAB).

Sometimes a baby's genitalia do not appear to be entirely male or female, and the baby is categorized as intersex. (See page 165 for more.) Some places allow intersex to be assigned on birth certificates, but even though around 1.7 percent of people have intersex variations, most parents and guardians still have to assign their child to the sex binary of male or female, despite the inexactness.

Hormones and Puberty

The sex you are assigned at birth has a lot to do with the type and amount of hormones your body produces. Hormones are chemicals that guide physical, mental, and emotional development throughout a person's entire life. Your body produces dozens of different hormones, but the main hormones this manual focuses on are the two primary sex hormones: testosterone and estrogen.

Testosterone and estrogen are called sex hormones because when you're a little kid, your body tends to not have many physical "male" or "female" traits. But once puberty starts (often between the ages of eight and fourteen), your sex hormones activate and mature your body in "male" or "female" ways.

The main male sex hormone is testosterone, produced by the testicles. Testicles produce just a little estrogen and a lot of testosterone. This combination leads to the development of "male" sex traits—the penis and testicles enlarge and darken, the voice deepens, facial and body hair increases, and muscle mass develops.

The main female sex hormone is estrogen, produced by the ovaries. Ovaries produce a little testosterone and a lot of estrogen. This combination leads to the development of "female" sex traits—hips and thighs widen, nipples and labia enlarge and darken, breasts develop, and menstruation begins (see page 148).

You might be excited to see how puberty changes (or changed, if you already went through it) your body into one that is more "masculine" or "feminine"—new body hair, a bigger butt, stronger muscles . . . or you might also feel annoyed, scared, or confused by what's going on, or have a combination of feelings. It's perfectly normal to swing back and forth between being happy or stressed or sad about everything that's happening to your body—as you can see from this manual, there's a whole lot going on with all of our bodies, and it can take some time to figure everything out!

Sometimes, however, your emotions about your developing body may feel more complex or intense. That's okay, too. Your feelings can be heavily influenced by a variety of factors, including your gender identity (see page 167).

Intersex Variations

An intersex variation is any type of hormonal, chromosomal, and/or genitalia development that doesn't fit neatly into the category of "male" or "female." Did you know that in the womb, the same tissue that labia develops from can also become the scrotum? And the clitoris and penis develop from the same tissue, too? Most of the time, a person is born with internal and external genitalia that are either 100 percent male or 100 percent female. However, people with intersex variations are born with a diverse combination of both.

Sometimes, intersex variations are noticed at birth because the infant's genitals appear not to be either a "penis" or "vulva" (as mentioned on page 164). Often, however, people with intersex variations are born with genitals that look like they are either "male" or "female," and they don't find out about their variations until later in life. For example, some people born with vaginas might learn that their internal genitalia are testicles instead of ovaries because they never start menstruating. Or a person assigned female at birth might realize over time that they were born with a very small penis that later becomes more obvious, especially after puberty activates their "male" hormones.

Indeed, not everyone is born with the kind of genitalia you'll see in most of the pictures in this manual, and *there is nothing wrong with that*. People's bodies are beautifully complicated and can have all sorts of variations (not just their genitalia), which means that most of us don't fit some set of expectations—either our own or someone else's. But a variation is not the same as ugly or unhealthy—it's just unique! In fact, most people with intersex variations are perfectly healthy, and the health problems they might have are usually unrelated to their genital diversity.

If you notice signs of intersex variation, see your doctor for screening and possible diagnosis and treatment (if desired). And consider talk therapy, which might help you sort out any feelings or emotions that may come up with such a discovery. See page 197 for more on caring for your mental health.

> There are millions of people with intersex variations around the globe! Worldwide, around 1.7 percent (and possibly more) of all people, according to many different scientific and advocacy sources. To put this number in perspective, around 2 percent of people worldwide are born with green eyes, up to 2 percent of people worldwide have vitiligo (see page 37), less than 1 percent of people worldwide have inflammatory bowel disease (page 114), up to 2 percent of the global population have red hair, and less than 1 percent of people under the age of twenty have juvenile diabetes.

When People Look At (and Treat) You Differently

Unfortunately, when other people notice your changing body, they may start treating you differently, and not always in ways you appreciate or that make you feel safe. Society tends to unfairly (and often incorrectly) refer to the physical you in order to make assumptions about the type of person you are and how to communicate with or about you. People might see your new body shape, facial hair, or height and assume you're a lot more tough, more sexual, or just overall more grown-up than you feel inside. This can feel frustrating at best and scary at worst. Know that you aren't imagining things, and that no matter your sex or gender, it's never okay to be made to feel uncomfortable in your own skin emotionally, verbally, or especially physically—see page 185 for advice on what to do if someone crosses your personal boundaries sexually. And as always, like with any issue, finding trusted people to talk to can help tremendously.

> Hijras in South Asia, muxes in Mexico, and the Māhū in Native Hawaiian culture are a few of the dozens of global examples of the many different genders that can be found in our very diverse world.

Gender Identity

Gender identity is how you feel about your gender internally: male, female, a combination of both, neither . . . or any of many (MANY) other gender identities! While your sex is assigned for you at birth, absolutely no one can tell you how "male" or "female" you feel inside (though some people might try). Likewise, you can't tell anyone else how they should feel, either—gender identity is extremely personal.

You can't just look at a person and assume to know their gender based on their appearance. That's why it's commonly said that "genitalia is what's between our legs, while gender is what's between our ears."

Most people's sex assigned at birth matches pretty closely with their gender identity. These people are cisgender. The prefix *cis* means "on this side"—meaning a cisgender person's gender and assigned sex are alike.

Sometimes there's a mismatch and a person's gender identity is not the sex they were assigned at birth. These people are transgender. The prefix *trans* means "on the other side of."

Dozens of other gender identities abound. The term *nonbinary* ("not just two") is a common way to simply identify as not either fully "male" or "female." An agender person doesn't identify with any gender (here, the prefix *a* means "without"). Other gender identities include being gender fluid, gender nonconforming, genderqueer, and more.

At the end of the day, we're all just people who deserve love, safety, and respect!

> Like everyone else, intersex people all have different ways of expressing their gender identity that may or may not socially match up with the sex they were assigned at birth.

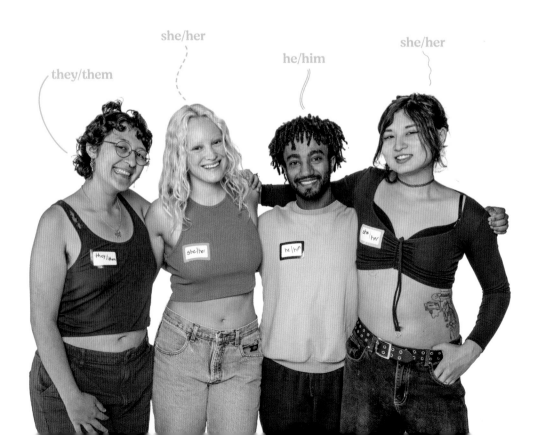

they/them   she/her   he/him   she/her

Ze, She, He, They (Pronouns)

Sharing your personal pronouns when you meet people (and asking for theirs) is a wonderful way to affirm gender. After our first name, our pronouns are the most common words people use to describe us. While many people are comfortable with their assigned-at-birth pronouns (he/him/his for males and she/her/hers for females), it's not uncommon to choose different personal pronouns that are a better fit, whether it's using "he" instead of "she" or something else. They/them/theirs is one of the most common gender inclusive alternatives, but there are others as well, including xe/xem/xyrs, ze/zir/zirs, or even "that one."

Gender Dysphoria

For many people, exploring their gender identity is an enjoyable process, but for other people it can be super stressful. If exploring your gender is an unpleasant experience filled with negative feelings like shame, loneliness, and dissatisfaction, you might be experiencing gender dysphoria, which is when there's a lot of stress and distress surrounding your gender identity.

Gender dysphoria doesn't show up only at puberty. People of all ages can find themselves in need of support to help unpack not just what's going on with themselves and their bodies but also the actions and reactions of other people in their school, home, work, and social lives. If you think you might have gender dysphoria or might just be feeling more overwhelmed than usual (we all do sometimes!), finding a professional with knowledge about gender dysphoria to talk about what's going on can really help. See page 198 for different types of therapists.

Express Yourself!

Whatever your gender, it can feel fun and empowering to make intentional choices about what you wear, how you style your hair, and even how you walk and talk. This is called gender expression. From wearing baggy jeans to spritzing yourself with floral perfume to using a binder to flatten your chest to applying lipstick, there are countless ways to evolve the external expression of your internal gender identity. Some people feel more comfortable expressing their gender only in private, and that's totally okay, too. You can also express yourselves in ways that break the norms of your gender; despite some common misinformation, there's no one "type" of person who is "supposed"

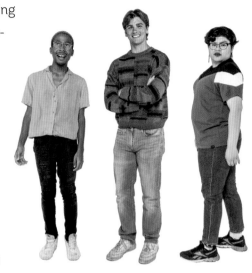

to do things like cry freely, fix cars, wear nail polish, play basketball, or any number of choices that are just that—choices. So choose what makes you feel whole!

If you're feeling overwhelmed by all this information, just remember:

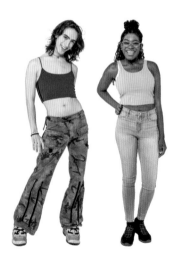

**Genitalia determine the sex
you are assigned at birth,**

but neither your genitalia

nor your sex

determines your gender.

Only YOU can identify your gender.

**That's why it's called
YOUR gender identity!**

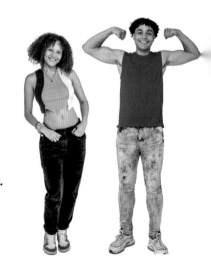

*These seven people were asked to come to the photo shoot
dressed in their favorite casual outfit—don't they all look great?*

Sometimes people use hormone therapy to increase their estrogen or testosterone levels in order to affirm their gender identity. People born with vaginas who produce or take more testosterone may find their voices deepen and facial hair increase. People born with penises who produce or take additional estrogen might see breast growth and thinner facial and body hair. (See page 164 for more on hormones.) Right now, access to gender-affirming care varies by age and location. However, every major North American medical organization, including the American Academy of Pediatrics, the American Psychiatric Association, the American Medical Association, and the Endocrine Society supports gender-affirming care for trans and gender-diverse youth.

Reproduction

Even though you might not *want* to have children, part of your body's maturation process is to develop so that, if desired, you can play a role in creating new people, a process formally known as reproduction.

Reproductive cells called gametes make reproduction possible. The gametes of people are eggs and sperm. Ovaries produce and store eggs, which are released as part of the menstrual cycle (more on this on page 148). Testicles produce and store sperm, which are ejaculated via semen (more on this on page 140). In order for people to reproduce and create more people, sperm must combine with an egg, either through sex or medical procedures. This combination creates an embryo, which can eventually grow into a baby. Every year, millions of babies are born, and each of them will, hopefully, spend a lot of time as they grow up trying to figure out who the best version of themselves is and how they can become it—just like you are doing right now.

Thanks to our unique menstrual cycle, humans are one of the few mammals that can reproduce year-round (instead of only seasonally, like horses and foxes).

Who Do You Love?

Always remember that a person's sex assigned at birth or a person's gender identity (see page 167) NEVER determines the type of person they're attracted to physically. That is called your sexual orientation. As your body develops during puberty, so does your sense of desire and sexuality. It's normal to find yourself "crushing" on people and thinking about them in a different, more romantic or sexual way than before.

Like gender, figuring out your sexual orientation can be a little complicated. You may be surprised by the type of people who, when you think about them, cause you to have a racing heartbeat, sweaty palms, spontaneous erections, a moist vagina, dry mouth, stammering voice, blank mind . . . it's incredible what attraction can do to the body and brain!

Here are some helpful descriptors to help you understand a few of the many types of sexual orientations, in alphabetical order:

✦ **Asexual.** Here, the prefix *a* means "without"—an asexual person tends to not feel much or any sexual attraction toward anyone.

✦ **Bisexual.** The prefix *bi* means "two"—a bisexual person can be sexually attracted to more than one gender.

✦ **Demisexual.** The prefix *demi* means "half"—a demisexual tends to only feel sexual attraction toward someone after an emotional bond is formed.

✦ **Heterosexual.** The prefix *hetero* means "other"—a heterosexual woman is sexually attracted to men, and a heterosexual man is sexually attracted to women. "Straight" is a common slang word to describe being heterosexual.

✦ **Homosexual.** The prefix *homo* means "same"—a homosexual woman is sexually attracted to women, and a homosexual man is sexually attracted to men. Women who are attracted to women are often described as "lesbians." "Gay" is a common slang word to describe someone who is homosexual or romantically attracted to the same gender.

✦ **Pansexual.** The prefix *pan* means "all"—a pansexual person can feel sexual attraction toward all people.

Not every person has the same level of comfort hearing or using some or all of these words to describe themselves or others, as many people have experienced people using these words negatively, either in person or in the media. Whether you choose to reclaim, avoid, or invent your own terms, your feelings are valid.

There are many (MANY) more ways to describe a person's sexual orientation (Queer! Heteroflexible! Omnisexual! Graysexual!). And sometimes the type of person someone desires romantically (for a meaningful emotional connection) can be different from their sexual orientation (who they would like to be sexually intimate with). So know that it's totally possible to be heterosexual but biromantic, or homosexual and aromantic. You know your body and brain best, and you'll figure it out!

When figuring all this out, you might prefer to describe yourself as on a spectrum that may or may not fluctuate. Or you may not feel like any of these descriptions fit who you are, you may not want to label yourself at all, or you may find it helpful to come up with your own, super-specific labels. All of this is totally okay! Don't stress yourself out trying to fit into an unnecessary box—just live your life and love who you want to love. However you identify (or don't identify), just know that who you are, whoever you like, and however you love is awesome and enough, and the world needs you to be YOU!

A Sexually Active Person's Checklist

No one should be sexually active until they're really, really, REALLY ready. Many people are sexually active by the time they're twenty years old, but lots of people don't have sex until they're in their thirties, forties, or ever—and that's totally okay. However, if you become sexually active, there are ten (yes, ten) important things to know:

1. **Consent is crucial.** Consent means giving or asking for permission, and consent is required before and during any type of sexual activity. Consent should be:

   ○ **Legal.** Check your state laws. The age a person can consent to having sex with another person, even someone their own age, differs by location.

   ○ **Enthusiastic.** Any hesitation, lack of eye contact, mumbling, or other signs of discomfort should be taken as a "NO," especially if the person is being encouraged to consent, despite seeming unexcited. If spoken aloud, consent should be a "yes," expressed with confidence. A more uncertain "maybe" or "sure" or silence should always be equated with a "NO." Nonspeaking people or people who speak a different language can express consent with enthusiastic nodding, sign language, or via alternative communication devices. When there's doubt or confusion, it's a "NO."

   ○ **Informed.** It's not consent if a person doesn't know the truth about the situation, like STI status or if someone says they're on birth control or using a condom and they're not.

   ○ **Reversible**. It's always okay to change one's mind at any time, and no reason needs to be given either in the heat of the moment or after. (See page 143 on blue balls and blue vulva to eradicate the untruth that stopping sexual activity is bad for the body.)

○ **Specific**. Just because someone agrees to one thing doesn't mean they consent to anything else—consent to hug, for example, doesn't give consent to kiss—specific consent needs to be given for all experiences.

○ **Clear-minded.** A sleeping person or a person under the influence of drugs or alcohol is NOT capable of receiving or giving consent.

Don't try to skip consent in the heat of the moment, and don't let someone else's enthusiasm override your own lack of interest in consenting. Never pressure anyone to have sex who doesn't want to (including yourself), and don't allow anyone to pressure you into having unwanted sex.

Keep reading for more information about what to do if anyone touches your body without consent, which is sexual assault.

2 **Never assault someone.** Many parts of this manual mention the importance of never forcing a sexual situation, either on yourself or another person. If it happens to you, you did not deserve it and it is not your fault. Turn to page 185 for more on sexual assault.

3 **Make sure that you're doing it for the right reasons.** Ask yourself:

○ Do I use sex to prove something or to feel loved or powerful?

○ Am I pressuring someone to have sex or am I being pressured to have sex?

○ Am I practicing unsafe sex out of spite or because I'd secretly like to have a baby or get someone pregnant?

If you answered "yes" to any of the questions above, talk to a nurse, therapist, doctor, or other trusted person.

4 **ALWAYS use protection during penetrative sex—and not just if a penis is involved!** STIs can be transmitted via fingers, toys, tongues . . . you name it. Gloves, condoms (external and internal), and dental dams are just some of the options available for over-the-counter purchase at most drugstores. Your partner (or you) might complain that sex feels better without using protection, and that's a common concern. Just ask this question: If sex with protection feels bad, how much worse would it feel to be diagnosed with an STI?

External condoms are the number one way to prevent STIs (and pregnancy when people born with penises have penetrative intercourse with people born with vaginas). But you've got to use them properly. See page 179 for instructions.

5 **Stay away if you see sores on your partner's genitalia or face.** Steer clear of any type of wound, rash, or bloody spot on or near any place you might touch or kiss, as it can be a sign of infection that could get passed along to you through skin-to-skin contact.

6 **Get STI testing before getting it on (and after, too).** Instead of ice cream or coffee, make a date to get tested for STIs together before going too far. Lots of STIs have zero visible signs or symptoms, so the only way to catch many of them before they damage your body is by testing. When you're sexually active, you and your partner(s) need to be tested anywhere from every three months to once a year, depending on your sexual history. If you want to test yourself or your partner for an STI or would like condoms or other forms of contraception (devices and medicine that prevent pregnancy), ask your primary care physician or gynecologist, or search online for your local county or city health department, as they can usually steer you in the right direction. If the first place you call can't help you, ask for a referral. No matter how scared, embarrassed, or alone you may feel, keep trying—there's *always* a place to go for help.

7 **Talk to your doctor about the HPV vaccine**. HPV is an STI that is often undetectable but is extremely easy to transmit via skin-to-skin contact, and while some types can clear up on their own, others can pose a serious threat to your health. Most people can get the vaccine to prevent HPV-related cancers and some strains of genital and anal warts.

Talk to your doctor about PrEP. PrEP (pre-exposure prophylaxis) is an injection or oral medication that, if taken properly, can eliminate nearly all cases of human immunodeficiency virus (HIV), an immune system disease that, if left untreated, can lead to more complicated diseases such as AIDS (acquired immunodeficiency syndrome). HIV is transmitted through sexual activity and injection drug use, so talk to your doctor to see if PrEP is right for you based on your sexual history and risk factors.

Pay close attention to your or your partner's cycles if you/they menstruate. You aren't just at risk for STIs but also for unplanned pregnancy. By keeping track of your/your partner's menstrual cycle (see page 151) and even vaginal discharge cycles (page 159), you can stay on top of your sexual health before an issue causes damage or becomes untreatable.

Have fun! If you're still interested in having sex after all this (LOL), don't forget to enjoy yourself! Can having sex be a pretty big decision? Absolutely. But once you've made the informed choice to do so, and you've put in the work to be fully prepared and comfortable, don't let all this important planning take away from the fact that responsible and consenting sex, *when you are ready*, can be an incredible (incredible!) experience! Enjoy the exciting process of figuring out what feels amazing and what doesn't. And don't be afraid to share your likes and dislikes—and encourage your partner to share, too. Keeping an open and honest line of communication is key to a healthy and happy relationship. And remember: sometimes talking about sex can feel as good as sex itself!

Speaking of Fun . . .

Sexual pleasure, like many aspects of this manual, is a deeply personal spectrum. Figuring out what feels good and what doesn't is a lifelong journey, and sometimes you might be surprised by what you do and don't enjoy. Some people like outercourse (see next section) more than intercourse; others hate the feeling of an orgasm but love a good massage. Solving your personal pleasure mysteries is part of the joy of being a human, as getting to have sex for pleasure is an evolutionary gift that doesn't appear to have been granted to all creatures. There's no "right" or "wrong" way to be sexually active, and you don't *have* to be sexually active at all. Just stay safe and respect your body and the bodies of others, and the rest will likely figure itself out along the way.

Outercourse

Don't forget that lots of fun can be had with a partner that doesn't involve genital-to-skin contact or the exchange of bodily fluids. Outercourse, such as rubbing clothed bodies together (also known as grinding or dry humping), fondling and massage, self-masturbating together, and using (but not sharing) toys instead of body parts can all be highly enjoyable and orgasmic experiences (sometimes better than intercourse!) that come with far less risk of pregnancy or STIs.

Types of Condoms (Always Use One!)

As of right now, aside from condoms, there are no options for people with penises to personally protect themselves and their partners from STIs. Condoms are also the only way for people born with penises to personally prevent pregnancy when having sex with people born with vaginas. Since toys can also transmit STIs from shared fluids, they should be covered in condoms when they're in use, too.

So, clearly, condoms are important! There are two types:

- **External condoms** are the condoms that are placed on the penis. It can be fun to try different sizes, shapes, flavors, and textures of condoms to find the one that's right for you or your partner.

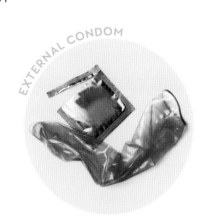

EXTERNAL CONDOM

- **Internal condoms** are inserted into the vagina or anus before penetration. They are useful alternatives to external condoms, especially when having sex with a person with a penis who "hates wearing condoms" (though that's never an excuse to not use them, especially if you've agreed to it—see page 174 for more on informed consent).

    They are sometimes called "female condoms," as they originated for people with vaginas, but they are now FDA approved for anal use also. While they are sold over the counter, they're often harder to find and are usually more expensive.

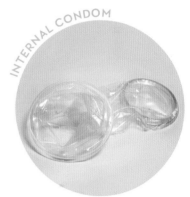

INTERNAL CONDOM

How to Properly Put a Condom on a Penis (No Teeth!)

After the penis becomes erect but before any physical contact with another person's mouth or genitals is the time to put on an external condom.

Some uncircumcised people find it easier to put the condom on after pulling their foreskin back.

When you're ready, putting on a condom is as easy as 1, 2, 3! Practice a few times when you're

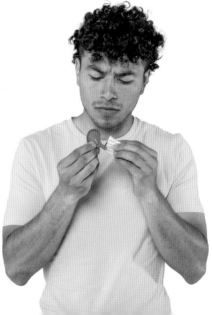

alone (either on your penis if you have one, or on a banana) so you're ready to (un)roll in the heat of the moment.

 STEP 1 Check to make sure the condom's not rolling inside out before putting it on—the top should look like a hat as it smoothly unrolls over the penis. This is the reservoir tip, where ejaculate (semen) collects. If you realize as you're unrolling that the condom is on wrong, take it off, throw it away, and start over, as the outside of the condom may have been exposed to STIs and sperm from the penis.

 STEP 2 Pinch the reservoir tip as you place the condom on the head of the penis to leave space for the semen.

 STEP 3 Roll the condom all the way down until it reaches the pubic hair and covers the entire penis.

Right after ejaculation, the person wearing the condom should use their fingers to hold it tight to their body to avoid semen spillage as they carefully withdraw before their penis becomes soft. Once safely withdrawn, the condom can then be removed and thrown away. Never flush condoms, or be prepared for a plumber's bill! Ready to go again? Use a new condom every time and have fun!

> One brand-new condom at a time, please! Don't think that "double bagging" condoms equals twice the protection. Two condoms actually cause friction, which can tear the material, enabling sperm and STIs to flow through.

Dental Dams

While a dental dam isn't a condom, this thin rectangle of latex is an easy-to-use and awesome way to prevent STIs during oral sex on a vulva or anus. If an "official" dental dam is not available, researchers believe that cutting open a latex condom or using household plastic wrap are better options than using no protection.

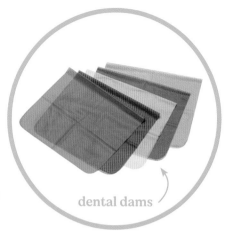

dental dams

> Permanent birth control, formally called medical sterilization, is a surgery that doctors can perform to forever prevent accidental pregnancy from sexual activity—usually in the form of vasectomies for people born with testicles and tubal ligation for people born with ovaries. However, medical sterilization doesn't protect against STIs, so condoms still need to be used. (FYI, people born with vaginas who are medically sterilized can often still get pregnant via medical procedures, and people born with penises often can have their sterilization reversed, though these procedures aren't guaranteed to work. See page 171 for more on reproduction.)

Additional Birth Control Options (to Use with Condoms!)

The following birth control methods are to be paired with condom usage to prevent people born with vaginas from getting pregnant. You must use condoms (can that be said enough?) because they are the best and easiest form of protection against STIs, but ideally no one should depend on them as their only form of birth control. Even when condoms are used correctly, their failure rate can be up to 13 percent. When teeth are used to rip open the package, if the condom isn't put on before semen begins to flow, if it's been sitting in a backpack for a few years, or if other infractions take place (like putting on two at once), the failure rate skyrockets.

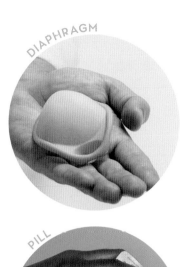
DIAPHRAGM

+ **The diaphragm.** Before genital contact begins, a silicone dome-shaped barrier is smeared with spermicide (more on page 184) and vaginally inserted by the user, where it stays for at least six hours after intercourse to prevent sperm from entering the cervix. Your doctor can give you a prescription for this nonhormonal form of contraception and help you learn how to insert yours properly. When used alone, diaphragms fail 17 out of every 100 users.

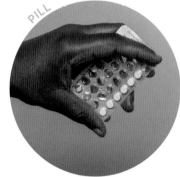
PILL

+ **The pill.** Every day at the same time, a pill is swallowed that contains pregnancy-preventing hormones. Sometimes the pills contain no hormones for one week out of the month, which is when menstruation occurs, and sometimes people take hormonal birth control pills continuously to avoid getting a period at all (if you'd rather not menstruate, talk to your doctor to see if this may be an option for you). With average use, meaning a pill is occasionally forgotten or taken late, birth control pills fail 7 out of every 100 users.

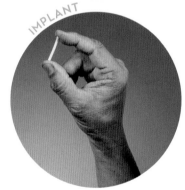
IMPLANT

+ **The implant.** Every few years, a tiny rod is implanted in the upper arm by a medical profes-

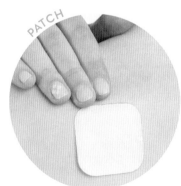
PATCH

sional, where it releases pregnancy-preventing hormones. The implant fails 1 out of every 1,000 users.

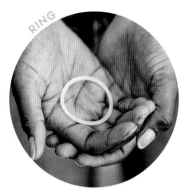

+ **The patch.** Once a week on the same day, for three weeks out of the month, an adhesive patch is applied to the stomach, arm, butt, or upper body by the user, where it releases hormones through the skin and into the bloodstream to prevent pregnancy. No patch is worn during the fourth week, which is when menstruation occurs. The patch fails 7 out of every 100 users.

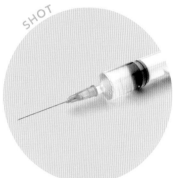

+ **The ring.** Once a month, a flexible plastic ring is inserted into the vagina by the user, where it stays for three weeks, slowly releasing pregnancy-preventing hormones. The ring is taken out during the fourth week, which is when menstruation occurs. The ring fails 7 out of every 100 users.

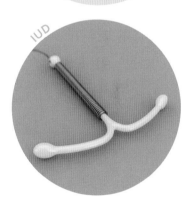

+ **The shot.** Every three months, a pregnancy-preventing hormone is injected by a medical professional into the arm or butt. The shot fails 4 out of every 100 users.

+ **The IUD.** Every few years, a small T-shaped device is placed inside the uterus by a medical professional, where it makes it difficult for sperm to fertilize an egg and also for fertilized eggs to implant in the uterus. There are hormonal and non-hormonal intrauterine devices (IUDs), each with different side effects, that your doctor can discuss with you. The IUD fails less than 1 out of every 100 users.

Spermicides are available for purchase over the counter, and while they are not effective enough to use alone, they are great to pair with other forms of contraception, like diaphragms and condoms. (Some condoms can be bought already covered in spermicide.) Before genital contact begins, a jelly, cream, pellet, foam, or film containing chemicals that slow down and kill sperm is vaginally inserted by the user, where it stays for at least six hours to prevent sperm from fertilizing an egg. When used alone, spermicides fail 21 out of every 100 users.

Emergency Contraception

If, for any reason, you had sex without protection or if the protection you tried to use failed (like if the condom broke), there are two forms of emergency contraception you or your partner can use to prevent pregnancy within five days of having unprotected sex.

+ **An IUD.** If you can get to a gynecologist or health clinic, having an IUD inserted within five days of having unprotected sex not only acts as emergency contraception but also serves as long-term contraception, so it's the best bet if you're planning on staying sexually active. It may or may not be covered by insurance or the clinic and could cost a couple of hundred dollars to have inserted, so check in advance and see if this would work for you.

+ **The "morning-after" pill.** The sooner the morning-after pill is taken after sexual intercourse, the more effective the medicine is in preventing pregnancy by impeding ovulation. Read directions carefully, as some types of pills may require taking them within three days of intercourse and others have a window of as many as five days. Some morning-after pills are sold over the counter in drugstores, and anyone of any age can buy them without a prescription. However, if you weigh over 165 pounds, you may need a prescription for a more effective version, so call your doctor or local health clinic immediately and be specific and honest about when you last had intercourse.

Spotting STI Spots

In the United States, 1 in every 5 people has a sexually transmitted infection, and half of all new STIs happen to people under the age of twenty-five. Remember to be careful and practice safe sex (see page 178) at all times, not just during vaginal or anal penetration. Oral sex and even kissing can spread many STIs, especially if there's an open sore on the mouth or genitalia. For example, rubbing another person's genitalia (either with your hands or your own genitalia) can easily spread warts and herpes without penetration.

Many STIs have similar symptoms (or none at all!), and only a doctor can identify which one you have. If you recognize any of the symptoms below, it's time to be tested.

- ✦ Any penile discharge that isn't urine, semen, or smegma
- ✦ A change in vaginal discharge
- ✦ Any anal discharge that's not poop
- ✦ Bumps, sores, or rashes in or on your genitalia or mouth
- ✦ Genital burning or itching
- ✦ Painful urination

Steps after Sexual Assault

Unfortunately, and unfairly, many people report being sexually assaulted at some point in their lives. Sexual assault includes unwanted sexual touching as well as rape, which is legally defined as penetration either of the anus or vagina for any duration of time, with any object or body part (including fingers and toys as well as penises), or orally by the sex organ of another person (like a penis) without the consent of the victim. (See page 174 for information on consent.)

Anyone can be sexually assaulted, regardless of sex, gender, or sexual orientation. Often the assaulter is someone the person knows. While no one wants to think about something like this happening either to themselves or a person they care about, it can and does happen. And if it does, or if it has, *DO NOT BLAME YOURSELF.* Sexual assault is never your fault, and it's important to protect yourself with the following steps after sexual assault:

+ **Get safe ASAP.** A hospital's emergency room is a good place to go immediately after an assault, as you can get care that includes medications to ward off STIs and other complications like pregnancy. Hospitals also usually have trained professionals available to help you report the sexual assault.

+ **Avoid brushing your teeth, bathing, or changing clothes.** A common first instinct might be to immediately wash away any trace of the assault, but not doing so gives the hospital a chance to carefully and respectfully collect evidence that could help identify or provide evidence against your attacker if you decide to pursue legal action. However, it's important to still seek medical care even if you have showered or changed. It's still often possible to capture certain types of evidence even days later, and preventative medication is still important to your long-term health.

+ **Seek mental health support.** Talk therapy should be immediately incorporated into your self-care routine as you process this traumatic event. Ideally, your mental health professional specializes in treating victims of assault, as assault victims may suffer from depression, turn to alcohol and drugs, or think about suicide. Talking to a trained professional or a support group on a regular basis can really help the healing process. See page 197 for more information on talk therapy and get the help and support you deserve.

No matter what, do not keep the assault to yourself—seek help ASAP. If you can't immediately get help in person, call or text the Suicide and Crisis Lifeline at 988 (see page 204 for more information) or call the Rape, Abuse, and Incest National Network (RAINN). They have a confidential 24/7 sexual assault helpline (1-800-656-HOPE) as well as an online hotline that can help you process this traumatic event and connect you to local support in your area.

seeking help & self-care

Always Seek Help!

Multiple times in life you will be faced with challenges and problems that you cannot solve on your own. You might even be going through something tough right now. When this happens, you can feel overwhelmed, scared, anxious, or unable to think straight, let alone seek help. It may feel easier to ignore concerns or try to deal with them alone, but don't. Always seek help from others as soon as possible, no matter how big or small the problem is. When in doubt, let it out!

Some common reasons you may find yourself needing to reach out for help include:

+ **Something looks or feels off with any part of your body—including your mind.** There are dozens of mental health professionals trained to help you understand and overcome any mental health problem, from depression to anxiety (page 200) to gender dysphoria (page 169) to post-traumatic stress disorder, or PTSD (page 201).

+ **Annual medical, eye, and dental wellness checks.** Getting a full-body checkup from a health professional at least once a year, including for your teeth and eyes, is important. That way, you can work on issues as soon as you notice them instead of waiting until they worsen and become more difficult to treat.

+ **You're having sex (or planning to soon).** A lot of responsibility goes along with having sex, and part of your self-care routine needs to involve professional help to get checked frequently for sexually transmitted infections (STIs) and to obtain the right birth control and STI protection for you. See page 185 for more on STIs and page 181 for information on prescription birth control.

Who Can Help You Seek Help?

If you need help immediately, like NOW, see page 204 for more information on contacting the Crisis Text Line or the 988 Suicide and Crisis Lifeline anytime, day or night.

There are dozens of people in your community and beyond who can help in the form of medical, mental health, and other types of assistance. If you're not sure what to do, a good first step is going to a responsible adult who knows you personally and whom you trust and feel comfortable talking to. Then look to other community leaders, like a teacher, school nurse, guidance counselor, faith leader, or social worker. Even if you don't have a community leader in particular that you're close to (or that even knows your name), these types of people are in positions of service, which means their profession is helping people just like you.

If you already have access to a doctor or therapist, reach out to them. (If you don't yet have a doctor or therapist, see page 192 for more on types of doctors and see page 198 for types of therapists.)

And as mentioned on page 196, if the first (or fourteenth) person you seek help from doesn't fit your needs, keep searching and get the help you need.

There Might Be Professional Help Online!

More and more medical professionals are offering online video and phone consultations (also known as telemedicine or virtual care), which can be helpful when seeking care for problems that don't necessarily require an in-person examination. For example, you can email some doctors a picture of a suspicious spot on your neck, and they'll respond back shortly with a diagnosis and send a prescription into your preferred pharmacy ASAP. (Not all issues can be addressed virtually, and depending upon your age you may need a caregiver to help navigate telemedicine.) Check to see if your healthcare providers offer this and if your medical insurance covers virtual care (see page 196 for more on medical costs).

> Many mental health professionals who offer talk therapy and medication are capable of doing so online.

Medical Professionals You Need Now

The three types of medical professionals you absolutely need to see at least once a year (see the self-care checklist on page 205) are a primary care practitioner (PCP), a dental health professional, and an eye health professional. If you have a vagina, a gynecologist should also eventually become part of your medical team.

- ✦ **Primary care practitioners (PCPs).** PCPs are perhaps the most common medical professionals in people's lives. You need to see your PCP once a year for an annual checkup, but any time you are dealing with a health issue, like allergies, a sexually transmitted infection, or depression, your PCP is someone you can call on for advice and medication.

  Once you've established a relationship with a PCP after an initial in-person checkup, you should be able to reach out to their office over the phone or online whenever you have a question or aren't feeling well. PCPs are great because if they can't help you with your specific problem, they can refer you to specialists who can. They also maintain a running history of your health so they can keep up with your health habits, any ongoing allergies or concerns, and help with long-term self-care goals.

  If you don't already have a PCP, it's time to find one. If you're a minor, you might need some help from the person who handles your healthcare.

  Many types of medical professionals can serve as your PCP:

  - ✦ **Medical doctors.** This includes pediatricians (who focus on people mostly under the age of eighteen), general practitioners, including doctors of family medicine (who take care of people of all ages), and internists, who focus on the body's internal organs and systems.

  - ✦ **Osteopathic doctors.** These doctors have additional training in a "whole body" medical approach that may utilize alternative, complementary, or non-Western medicine.

- **Physician assistants.** PAs have less training than medical doctors but can provide quality care, and they often work under the guidance of medical doctors.

  - **Nurse practitioners.** These professionals are skilled at managing patient care and may work alone or with a medical doctor.

- **Dental health professionals.** They treat and prevent problems with your gums, mouth, and teeth. Ideally, you see a dental health professional every six months to prevent small, common problems like cavities from turning into major problems like root canals and tooth loss. At the dentist's office, hygienists (who clean your teeth) and technicians (who help make braces, dentures, and other hardware) may aid the dentist. In addition, some communities have dental therapists and other professionals who travel around to schools, hospitals, and other local places to offer free or low-cost oral healthcare for people who otherwise couldn't afford dental work. If you or your family is unable to make an appointment with the dentist because of cost, your school counselor might have suggestions, or you can call local dentists in your area and ask if they know of any resources, such as a local dentistry school that offers free or low-cost services.

- **Eye health professionals.** They make sure your eyes are healthy, check your eyesight is clear, and provide you with eyeglass and contact prescriptions and therapies if needed. Seeing the optometrist or ophthalmologist once a year is important because if your eyesight is off, other aspects of your health can be affected, too. Eye health professionals often have no- or low-charge events in certain locations (like at school or in a shopping center), so be sure to check what services are available in your community.

- **Gynecologists/obstetricians.** Ob-gyns take care of the reproductive systems of people with vaginas. Annual visits to the gynecologist are recommended in order to get pelvic exams and other routine tests, as well as to help with period problems, sexually transmitted infections, vaginal infections and pain, breast issues, and prescriptions for birth control. Some gynecologists are also obstetricians who provide care for pregnant people and deliver babies. Many PCPs can perform the same types of checkups and prescribe the same medicines that gynecologists do, so you might want to ask yours if they can do double duty before seeking out a separate doctor.

When you're shopping in a store that sells prescription medicine, the pharmacist is usually available to answer questions about over-the-counter medication, too, so don't be afraid to ask about anything from jock itch cream to the morning-after pill! If you stumble upon a pharmacist who is less than helpful, don't give up on your health needs and goals! Try calling around to different pharmacies until you get the advice that you need.

Medical Professionals You Might Need

Specialists are medical professionals who focus their education and training on a specific area of medicine or surgery. Medical specialists probably won't be doctors you see every year, but there may be times in your self-care journey when they play a big role. Your PCP can often refer you to these types of specialists, or you can make an appointment directly.

+ **Allergists** screen for and treat things like asthma, immune diseases, and allergies to pets, pollen, dust, mold, and foods.

+ **Cardiologists** screen for and treat conditions involving the heart and other parts of the circulatory system.

+ **Dermatologists** screen for and treat conditions that affect the skin, nails, hair, and sweat glands.

+ **Endocrinologists** screen for and treat conditions involving the body's hormonal system, like diabetes. They also can specialize in gender-affirming hormone therapy.

+ **Gastroenterologists** screen for and treat conditions involving the digestive system, like constipation and vomiting.

+ **Neurologists** screen for and treat conditions involving the nervous system, like brain tumors.

+ **Oncologists** screen for and treat cancer.

+ **Orthopedists** screen for and treat conditions involving bones, muscles, and joints.

+ **Otolaryngologists (also known as ENTs)** screen for and treat conditions involving the ears, nose, and throat.

+ **Physical therapists** screen for and treat conditions involving pain or mobility by using specialized exercises and other therapies.

+ **Podiatrists** screen for and treat conditions involving the feet, ankles, and lower limbs.

+ **Radiologists** screen for all sorts of conditions using X-rays, ultrasounds, CT scans, PET scans, and MRI scans of your body.

+ **Surgeons** treat conditions by repairing, removing, or replacing body parts.

+ **Urologists** screen for and treat conditions involving genitalia and the urinary system.

Finding Help You Can Trust

If you have a gender, physical, or mental health concern and find that when you try to discuss it with others, no one seems to believe you or wants to engage in a conversation about it, try not to be surprised or take it personally. Some people (even professionals) may not want to get involved because they know they do not have the language or training necessary to help. Others may not believe your issues are serious, unfortunately. Some people are hesitant to automatically assume that a problem they can't see is real. They may first think that you're too young to be having these types of problems or that you're exaggerating or being dramatic.

Don't give up if the first person you reach out to doesn't end up being a right fit . . . or even the second . . . or the fourth. It can take time and patience to find a good and trustworthy care team, so keep trying until you get the right help that you need. If you're pretty clear about the issues you need help with, seek specific people and organizations that may specialize in helping people with those issues, like a clinic that specializes in LGBTQ+ health, a dermatologist who specializes in hyperpigmentation on African American skin, or a therapist who specializes in OCD. Sometimes it helps to spread your search for personalized care as far as your insurance will cover, even if it means not seeing someone locally (see page 191 for information on virtual care). It might be a little extra effort, but it's worth it to possibly get more targeted care!

Remember that you have a right to medical professionals who are available, caring, respectful, and aware of what you need, so don't be afraid to switch clinics and teams until you find support that you trust and respect and that trusts and respects you in return.

Medical Costs and Health Insurance

Because the American healthcare system is tangled up in everything from household income to age to employment, it can be difficult to find medical professionals who will treat you if you don't have the right kind of health insurance or cash to pay up-front. This difficulty can cause shame about your situation and concern about medical bills, which might make you or your family want to put off seeing the doctor or dentist, leading to worsening health problems.

Don't feel bad about something you have no control over! If you are under the age of nineteen, there is a good chance you can get a free or low-cost health insurance plan that will help you get the care you need. Even if you can't get health insurance, many areas offer free or low-cost health services at clinics, especially regarding sexual health. Just ask around until you find the help you need, because you deserve it.

Caring for Your Mental Health

While self-care (like the suggestions that start on page 205) can go a long way in looking after your mental health, sometimes you need some extra support from a professional. Mental health professionals help diagnose and treat behavioral and emotional issues (see page 199 for a list of common concerns). But they aren't just important in times of crisis (though they are invaluable then). It's a great idea to talk to a therapist or other mental health professional, even when things are going okay, so that when you have a problem and you need to talk about it, the therapist already knows you and a little bit about your story.

There are two main ways mental health professionals can help—talk therapy and medication. Many personal wellness plans include either one or both.

Talk Therapy

Talk therapy, formally known as psychotherapy, is all about learning how your mind works and helping you go after the life that you want. During talk therapy, a trained mental health professional can help you work through all kinds of emotional issues, problematic behaviors or thoughts, depression, anxiety, substance abuse, and other concerns. Talking to a professional can be more helpful than just chatting with friends and family, because you might feel more comfortable opening up to someone who isn't directly part of your life (especially if your issues have to do with your friends and family). While your social circle may be supportive, they might not have the tools to give good advice or help you come up with coping strategies, which a licensed mental health professional has obtained over many years of education and training.

Talk therapy can be in a one-on-one setting or in a group. Online talk therapy using a phone, computer, or other device has been shown to be very effective, especially for people with transportation issues or who live in areas with few mental health providers.

Some common types of licensed professionals that provide talk therapy include:

+ **Therapists.** Qualified to provide people with short- and long-term support, counseling, and guidance, therapists must hold a master's degree, medical degree, or doctorate-level qualification in one of a variety of fields, including counseling, psychiatry, social work, and clinical psychology. Check to see if your school or college has a therapist in-house to support student mental health. If so, speak with them about your problems, and if they can't help you directly, ask them for a community provider recommendation.

+ **Clinical social workers.** Therapists who are also trained in helping people access community resources, such as nutrition assistance programs.

+ **Psychologists.** Therapists who hold a master's degree or doctorate-level qualification specifically in psychology and are licensed to clinically diagnose people with specific problems and disorders.

Mental Health Medication

Your therapist may suggest you consider medication to help with your mental health journey. Medication can be very helpful in managing specific emotional or behavioral issues, either temporarily or long term. However, mental health medications must be prescribed only after consulting a trained medical professional to make sure the medicine will work for your specific issues. Never take someone else's prescribed medication, even if they say they have the same issue you think you do. Not everyone reacts the same way to prescription medicines, and only your doctor can make sure that you aren't allergic or don't have a personal history that could negatively interact with the medication.

Therapists and psychologists can't legally prescribe or recommend medications unless they are also licensed to do so. While your PCP has the ability to prescribe many mental health medications, like antidepressants, depending upon your treatment needs they or your therapist might refer you to a psychiatrist.

Psychiatrists are medical doctors with many years (usually around a decade) of training, specifically in mental health. They are also qualified to help with more complex issues, such as gender dysphoria, substance abuse issues, suicidal ideation, obsessive-compulsive disorders, and more. While a psychiatrist does not usually practice talk therapy, as part of their evaluation to determine which medication (if any) might be best for you, they will ask you multiple questions, and they may also consult with your therapist or PCP.

Nurse practitioners and physician assistants who specialize in psychiatry often work under the supervision of, or in collaboration with, a psychiatrist. In these capacities they, too, can prescribe mental health medication.

Common Mental Health Issues

The best thing about having a mental health professional on your self-care team is that they can be there for you if (when) you are struggling more than usual. Changing hormones in your teens and early twenties can cause your mental health to be especially fragile. Currently, more than 1 in 5 adult Americans are living with a mental health condition, and 1 in 5 teens will be diagnosed with a serious mental illness at some point during their lifetime.

Depression and anxiety are two of the most common mental health conditions, both of which often coexist together and can be treatable with professional help.

Signs of Depression and Anxiety

✦ **Depression.** Unshakable feelings of sadness, emptiness, irritability, or disinterest in everything and everyone around you are common symptoms of depression. Depression can also (but not always) make it difficult to sleep or get out of bed and to perform basic tasks like brushing teeth or going to school. There are many types of depression, with different signs and symptoms, and some people have more than one. A medical professional can screen and assess the best type of help for your needs.

✦ **Anxiety.** Unshakable feelings of fear and danger that cause intense emotional reactions, such as panic, are common symptoms of anxiety. Anxiety can also make it difficult to go places, interact with people, or take on responsibilities. Sometimes even thinking about doing certain things can bring on an uncontrollable and life-interrupting anxiety attack. There are many types of anxiety disorders, with different signs and symptoms, and some people have more than one. A medical professional can screen and assess the best type of help for your needs.

Sometimes mental health issues like depression and anxiety are temporary due to hormones, medications, current life circumstances, or a specific one-time event, but often they are longer-term conditions that are important (and possible) to manage throughout your life with the right outside support. See page 197 for advice on how to care for your mental health with talk therapy and possibly medication.

When You "Don't Look" Depressed or Anxious

While it's true that many people with depression or anxiety find it difficult or even impossible to perform basic daily survival tasks, that's not always the case. Some people have depression or anxiety symptoms (or symptoms of both) even while accomplishing impressive goals, but that doesn't mean that they don't need or deserve help. In fact, this is a common reason why many "high-achieving" people put off getting treatment, even when they feel like they're just going through the motions and not enjoying any of the successes. If you're simultaneously achieving goals but mentally in a hole, seeking help is okay—and important.

Other Mental Health Conditions to Know

✦ **Obsessive-compulsive disorder (OCD).** When you repeat a cycle of reoccurring thoughts (obsessions) and behaviors (compulsions) over and over again. OCD tends to ramp up over time, so if you notice habits forming that you can't control and are causing problems for you, talking to a mental health professional early on can be very helpful to get things under control before they become disruptive to your life. Some issues discussed in this manual, like hair-pulling disorder (see page 66), are on the obsessive-compulsive spectrum.

✦ **Post-traumatic stress disorder (PTSD).** When a person survives an extremely difficult situation or witnesses an especially distressing occurrence (whether in person or through the media), sometimes it becomes very tough or even impossible to recover from that experience. PTSD can also cause people to feel empty, hopeless, like they can't trust anyone or anything, or extremely anxious. An accident, violence, neglect, and death of a loved person or pet are all traumas that can trigger PTSD symptoms like avoidance, nightmares, and involuntarily reliving the experience. About 6 percent of the population will have PTSD at some point in their lives.

✦ **Body dysmorphic disorder (BDD).** When your body image is distorted and you obsess and fret over one or some of your features and traits to the point that many facets of your health are negatively impacted. Some of the issues discussed in this manual, such as bigorexia (obsession with muscles; see page 77), are types of BDD.

✦ **Eating disorders.** When constant negative thoughts and emotions about food, weight, or your body cause you to have difficulty eating nutritiously, putting your body at risk for malnourishment and other health issues. Any person of any gender or size can suffer from an eating disorder—it is not just a "girl" or "thin" person's disease. Eating disorders are more likely to start in the teens and early twenties, though they can begin at any time. The three most commonly known eating disorders are binge-eating disorder (also referred to as BED), bulimia (officially known as bulimia nervosa), and anorexia (known as anorexia nervosa). Binge-eating disorder is when a person eats lots of food in short periods of time, often in secret and even when not hungry. Bulimia is when a person binges on a lot of food quickly and then tries to purge it from their body using exercise, vomiting, food restriction, or laxatives. Anorexia is when a person severely restricts their food intake for fear of weight gain, even if they are dangerously underweight.

Other eating disorders include avoidant restrictive food intake disorder (ARFID), which is when a person restricts the amounts and types of food they consume, but not because of their body image (and sometimes in co-occurrence with autism or another disorder), and orthorexia, which is an obsession with healthy eating severe enough to disrupt day-to-day life.

If you feel you have an issue with your food intake that doesn't quite fit these descriptions, you may have what is called other specified feeding or eating disorder (OSFED). Talk to your doctor, who can help you get the care you need.

✦ **Substance abuse disorder.** When you lack the ability to control your impulse to smoke, drink alcohol, or use drugs, even though you know it's terrible for your health, and you may want to stop. More than 1 out of every 7 Americans over the age of twelve have a substance abuse disorder.

✦ **Attention-deficit/hyperactivity disorder (ADHD).** When you suffer from a cycle of one or all of the following in a way that makes day-to-day functioning difficult: hyperactivity (constantly moving), impulsivity (acting without thinking), and inattention (forgetfulness). Around 13 percent of teenagers are estimated to have had an ADHD diagnosis.

✦ **Self-harm.** When you injure yourself on purpose, not as a means to end your life but as a way to try to deal with stress, sadness, anger, and other intense emotions. Self-harm is a symptom of having a mental health issue and is estimated to affect almost 1 in 5 people worldwide and up to 30 percent of teens. The actual number is unknown, as most people who self-harm do it privately and feel too ashamed to seek professional help, despite it being very common.

If you see signs of yourself in any of these descriptions, talk to your doctor ASAP. Things can get better when you have the right people helping you.

Suicidal Thoughts

Always remember that your life is worth living. If you don't feel good, *seek help*. Never give up on yourself, and NEVER stop fighting for your health and well-being!

The number of people under the age of twenty who are at risk of suicide, meaning they are seriously considering ending their own life, is on the rise. More than 20 percent of high school students have seriously thought about suicide, so if you're one of them, you are not alone, and it's important to get the help and care you need.

Suicidal thoughts can be a condition of depression, anxiety, and other mental health conditions, and speaking with a trained professional can help you feel hope and get treatment, both in the moment and long term.

Let someone know when you're having suicidal thoughts—a trusted adult, a healthcare professional, or if you're in the United States, reach out to any of the following resources:

+ **For non-immediate needs, remember that 988 can be great.** Even if you don't need someone to immediately come to your location but you are having suicidal thoughts or are otherwise in need of mental health help, calling or texting 988 or speaking with a trained counselor at www.988lifeline.org can help manage emotional struggles. The counselor will listen carefully, try to understand what's going on, and offer support, coping strategies, and possible resources. Approximately 1 out of every 50 calls requires outside intervention, which means that 49 out of every 50 people are able to get the help they need from 988 without the involvement of law enforcement, an ambulance, or other emergency services.

◆ **Text 988 if calling is not an option for safety or capacity reasons.** Anyone can text 988, which is the 988 Suicide and Crisis Lifeline, and reach a trained counselor. Text support is currently available in English and Spanish. Usually, emergency services can be dispatched to your location if needed.

◆ **Chat via www.988lifeline.org/chat if you cannot or do not want to text or call for help.** Anyone can type in this URL and communicate via the Internet with a trained counselor in either English or Spanish. If it is determined that emergency services are needed, they can usually be dispatched to your location.

◆ **Call 911 and ask for an ambulance if you or someone you are with needs immediate, in-person help for their physical health or personal safety.** Almost anyone in the United States (and many people around the world) can call 911 to get emergency services like an ambulance to your location as soon as possible. The 911 phone support in the United States is available in many languages, including TTY communication for people who are speech disabled, deaf, or hard of hearing.

In an immediate crisis that's not necessarily mental health related? People experiencing any type of crisis (not just mental health related) can also contact the Crisis Text Line 24/7 to get information and emotional support. They can be reached on WhatsApp by messaging 443-SUPPORT (English) or 442-AYUDAME (Spanish), via chat at www.crisistextline.org, or by texting "HELLO" (English) or "HOLA" (Spanish) to 741741.

Being Self-Care Aware

Self-care is the lifelong process of making good decisions to keep your body and mind as healthy as possible.

Self-care doesn't just happen—every single day you must actively choose to put your health first, from drinking water instead of soda to showering regularly and going to sleep at a decent hour (instead of staying up and scrolling all night). Reading this manual and learning more about how you can take care of yourself is a form of self-care!

To that point, here's a checklist of some self-care actions you can take to put yourself and your health first. WARNING—it's a pretty long checklist! But don't worry—once you get into a good self-care routine, good habits start to form quickly, and all the tasks and reminders just become part of living your best life. Let's be real: you won't always feel up to checking off everything on the list, every single day—none of us do. Just try to stay on top of what you can, which is always good enough.

Your Self-Care Checklist

✦ **Use social media wisely.** When used properly, social media can be an amazing tool for people who are seeking support and solidarity that's difficult to find locally, especially when it comes to specific topics like unique hobbies, gender identity, medical issues, and more. That said, studies show the less social media you use, the better mental health and body image you have, and screen addiction is real and increasingly more common. Strive to sleep away from your screens at night, and whenever possible, replace the unhelpful social media scrolling and 24/7 texting with social activities, hobbies, and life goals. And make sure, to the best of your ability, that the people you follow and admire on social media are expressing views and sharing information that is factual, positive, and useful. Unfollow anyone spouting untruths or being negative or nasty (to themselves or toward others). If something you're scrolling by makes you feel worse after watching, block the account!

- ✦ **Sleep enough.** As hard as it may seem to go to bed early, getting between eight and ten hours each night has been proven to improve mood, physical health, and more. Nearly 3 out of every 4 teens don't sleep eight hours a day, but sleep is crucial to your health. Turn to page 208 for some tips to improve your time to snooze.

- ✦ **Exercise daily.** Thirty minutes a day of movement (walking counts!) is crucial to your self-care. (If you're a teenager, strive for an hour of exercise intense enough to make it difficult to talk.) Exercising strengthens your body and releases endorphins, which are hormones that can make you feel amazing, even when times are tough. You don't have to do the entire amount all at once—consider taking short movement breaks throughout the day to get in all the necessary minutes. And if you have a disability that makes exercise difficult, talk to your doctor about the best options for your specific capacities.

- ✦ **Clean yourself.** Daily bathing, toothbrushing, and wearing clean clothes can make a world of difference when it comes to how you feel physically and to your self-esteem.

- ✦ **Have hobbies and goals.** From learning a new language to solving a Rubik's Cube in sixty seconds or fixing a broken computer, creating purpose in your life with goals, fun activities, and interesting pursuits can give you something to look forward to and a reason to take care of yourself, even during difficult times.

- ✦ **Prevent injury.** You can't prevent every single accident, but being careful with your body is an important part of self-care. Some easy ways to avoid injury include scheduling and attending your annual checkups (see page 192), wearing sunscreen (page 30), putting on your seatbelt when in a car, and wearing a helmet when on a bike or scooter. Taking it a step further and refusing to do dangerous things like having unsafe sex (page 178), getting a tattoo from an unlicensed person (page 34), or trying a popular but risky social media challenge are also excellent additions to your self-care checklist. Remember, as I said at the beginning of this manual, this is the only body you'll ever get, so try to make it last!

- **Avoid smoking, alcohol, and drugs.** Vaping, drinking alcohol, and taking drugs can really mess with your mind and body—especially when you're in your teens. Sometimes the damage from abusing these substances when you're young can be permanent, so steer clear. If you've already started using, there's no better time to stop than now, but it might take help. A talk therapist who specializes in substance abuse is a great source of support if you want to or are using in order to feel good, fit in, or forget trauma. Turn to page 202 for more on substance abuse and page 197 for more on talk therapy. No matter how many of your friends or people in your community make it seem like no big deal, you don't have to be a statistic!

- **Don't take medications from other people.** Overdoses are on the rise, and that tiny pill someone says can make you feel better in a few minutes could very well be a more powerful prescription or illegal drug that can come with nasty side effects or even kill you within an hour. Even if someone tells you it's just a regular over-the-counter medicine, unless it comes in securely sealed packaging, politely decline.

- **Manage stress.** Easier said than done, but it's important and healthy to find ways to manage your stress. Some suggestions include exercise, eating well, doing yoga, or meditating.

- **Consume carefully.** The phrase "you are what you eat" is annoying but accurate. If you frequently skip meals or get your nutrition mostly from foods high in added sugar and simple carbohydrates (also known as processed foods), you might be hurting both your mental and physical health. It's been proven that drinking mostly water and eating lots of high-fiber foods (see page 102), fruits, and vegetables improve mood, gut health, and overall well-being.

- **Talk to trusted friends, adults, and medical professionals.** A huge part of self-care is surrounding yourself with kind, trustworthy people who can provide support and guidance if you're struggling with your physical or mental health. Don't hold whatever's hurting your body, mind, or soul inside! If you don't yet have anyone you feel comfortable talking to, it's time to find them.

> While this self-care checklist is pretty long, it's impossible to list every single thing that might help you take care of yourself, in part because every person is unique and has different needs. What are some things that you think could help you best care for your body and mind? Add 'em to your list!
>
> _____   _____
>
> _____   _____

Sleep Can Save Your Life

The clinical phrase "sleep hygiene" sounds weird, but it kind of makes sense: just like you have to bathe every day or else you *smell* funky, you need to get at least eight hours of sleep every night or else you *feel* funky! While eight hours of sleep may seem like an impossible goal considering all the stuff you have going on in your life (where is the time?!), trust that making time for good sleep will result in a smoother and more productive day. A well-rested mind can do homework faster (and more accurately), think more clearly and less impulsively (avoiding conflict), boost your mood (life is great!), and more. Studies have also shown that better sleep can improve symptoms of anxiety, depression, stress, and even more complicated mental health issues.

If you're struggling with insomnia (the inability to sleep), having a hard time falling or staying asleep, or just generally on the sleep struggle bus, consider rearranging your schedule for a month or two to make getting eight hours of sleep every night a top priority, and see if that helps. Here are some tried-and-true suggestions to help lead the way to Snoozetown:

- ✦ **Tell people you gotta sleep (for real).** Whether it's people who are used to texting you at all hours of the night, your family watching a movie, or your teacher assigning way too much homework, if other people are interfering with your ability to sleep, talk to them about it.

✦ **Kick your phone out of bed.** Even if it's your alarm clock, it can work just as well (or even better) across the room where you can't reach for it. Studies have proven that sleeping with your phone near your pillow messes with your sleep. And likely you'll be lucky to have missed some of the late-night online drama you might wake up to. So stow your phone away; you'll survive . . . and probably thrive!

✦ **Get comfy.** Is your pillow pitiful? Do you just fall asleep in the clothes you wore all day? You deserve better. If it's possible (and it isn't for everyone), a good quality pillow can be purchased for around twenty dollars. And switching out of clothes and into soft pajamas signifies to your body that it's time to wind down. If you haven't got any pajamas, or if you prefer to sleep in clothes, consider showering and sleeping in the clothes you're planning to wear the next day so that at least you're clean . . . and that's one less thing you'll have to do in the morning, meaning you can sleep longer!

✦ **Cancel out noise and light.** Sleep masks, earplugs, white noise videos or machines . . . whatever it takes to block out these common sleep stressors.

✦ **Get into a routine.** If your body starts to expect sleep, you sleep better. Commit to, if possible, going to bed and waking up around the same time every day. Even if you can't keep a consistent bedtime, daily nighttime rituals like taking a shower and putting on body lotion, fluffing your pillow and straightening out your blankets, meditating, or doing any other calming activity can trigger tiredness in your brain (and are also fun).

✦ **Trust the process.** It can take time for a new routine to set in, and the first week or so is often rocky, whether it's an exercise plan or a sleep schedule. You might just lie in bed for a bit the first few days, wondering if focusing on sleep is a terrible idea, but chances are if you keep at it, you'll find your sleep eventually improves.

✦ **Seek professional help if needed.** If you truly can't fall or stay sleep, you're not alone. Many people of all ages suffer from insomnia. If you can't fall or stay asleep no matter what you try, see your doctor. They can listen to your concerns, screen for any underlying issues that could be affecting your sleep (like restless leg syndrome), and possibly offer treatment solutions to help.

> Puberty messes with sleep, too! As you get older, the time of night when you start getting tired can become later by a few hours. Practicing good sleep habits can help you overcome your body's accidental internal efforts to sabotage your sleep.

Restless Leg Syndrome Is Real

Have you ever been in bed, relaxing or sleeping, and then all of a sudden, AAH! There's a strange sensation in one or both of your legs that causes a crawling feeling, or is itchy or painful? Sometimes you even need to get out of bed and walk around to try to get rid of the feeling, even if it's in the middle of the night. You aren't imagining things and you may have restless leg syndrome. More than 8 percent of teens and young adults have RLS. While sometimes confused with "growing pains," RLS is more severe and persistent.

> There are many other sleep-related disorders that young people suffer from that may warrant a visit to their doctor (or dentist) to discuss, such as tooth grinding and sleep paralysis. If your sleep isn't restful, it's important to get to the bottom of why!

If you can't kick your restless leg concerns after a week or two, see your doctor. They can screen for common issues that factor into the diagnosis of RLS, which include smoking, drinking alcohol or caffeine, and, ironically, sleep deprivation. They can also suggest treatment to help alleviate the symptoms.

Don't put a perfectionist spin on all this self-care. Some wise people say that "anything worth doing is also worth half doing." No one can do everything on this list all the time, the "right" way, no matter how hard you might want to. That's okay! Just do the best that you can and you'll see benefits.

final word:

be kind
to
yourself!

Let's keep it real: being a person is complicated. Change can be difficult. Accidents may happen and challenges will certainly be faced. So give yourself a break! Cut yourself some slack! Yes, it's easier said than done (speaking as someone who is especially hard on herself), but staying kind to yourself can really help you not just survive but thrive.

Throughout my life, I've been called all kinds of things: gorgeous, ugly, brilliant, ignorant, fabulous, foolish, great, gross . . . the list goes on and on. But in terms of affecting my self-esteem and self-worth, NOTHING matters as much as the words I say to or think about myself. Someone once told me never to talk to myself in a way I wouldn't let anyone else talk to me. That really stuck with me as an important part of my self-care journey.

Positive self-talk can help a lot with self-kindness, even when you're not feeling especially positive about anything or anyone, including yourself. So give it a try— what's the worst that could happen?

Whether in a whisper, in a shout, via sign language, using an alternate communication device, through journaling, or however you prefer to communicate, try telling yourself some (or all) of these phrases:

I AM WORTHY! I'M DOING MY BEST! I BELIEVE IN ME!

I AM MORE THAN ENOUGH! I'M A GOOD PERSON!

I AM STRONG! I'M GONNA FIGURE THINGS OUT!

(Because you totally are.)

about the author

Nancy Redd (she/her) is a loving wife and devoted mother of two kids (see page ix for why that's especially important for *The Real Body Manual*). She is also an award-winning *New York Times* and *USA Today* bestselling author and a Harvard-educated health journalist with almost two decades of experience. Nancy's super proud of the books she's written in a variety of genres, all with the fundamental goal of helping adults, young adults, and children understand, respect, and ultimately fall in love with themselves and their incredible bodies. Her most recent books include *Bedtime Bonnet*, the first-ever picture book to focus exclusively on Black nighttime hair rituals, written with the goal of encouraging healthy hair habits in her daughter (it worked!).

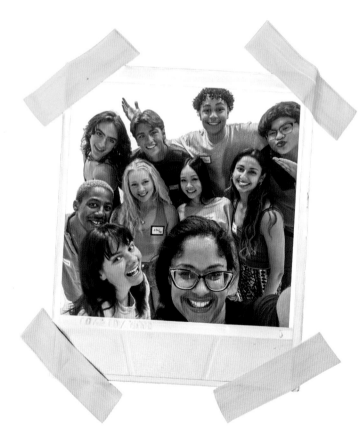

As you can see from this selfie, we had so much fun shooting the pictures for this manual! These are just some of the fantastic people who showed up to shoot with me (in the glasses) and my amazing photographer (the person next to me with the bangs)! Some came just to show off their great smiles, some came just to be part of the genitalia photos, and some came for it all, but EVERYONE'S contribution made a world of difference in making this manual really, really real.

acknowledgments

First off, a HUGE thank you to EVERYONE who picks up this book and reads even a single page—I hope you enjoy it and learn a lot! I'm the luckiest author in the world to have Hannah Steigmeyer as my remarkable editor . . . Hannah, you've been a delight to work with—it was love at first Zoom! And of course I'm also super grateful to the entire wonderful and supportive team at Avery, including awe-inspiring designer Ashley Tucker, brill production editor Leah Marsh, sharp copyeditors/proofreaders Meg Gerrity, Nancy Inglis, Claire Sullivan, and Jeanne Tao, powerhouse publicists Casey Maloney, Lillian Ball, and Chloe Boulard, and magical marketers Farin Schlussel and Neda Dallal. Also, huge thank you to Avery's former publisher Megan Newman, my current awesome publisher Tracy Behar, and last but not least, thank you to the gracious and savvy Lindsay Gordon, who I am honored to have known since we first started working together in 2010—can't believe we're all grown up now with our OWN kids!

In alphabetical order, thank you to my phenomenal and eagle-eyed medical experts who read and commented on different parts of this manual's text, pertinent to their expertise, including: Makunda Abdul-Mbacke, M.D., M.P.H., FACOG, who is a gynecologist; Christina B. Ching, M.D., who is a pediatric urologist; Katharine B. Dalke, M.D., MBE, who is a psychiatrist; Jennifer Gruenenfelder, M.D., who is a urologist; my very first reader Paria Hassouri, M.D., who is a pediatrician; Howard Leizer, PhD, who is a psychologist; Vinod Easwaran Nambudiri, M.D., MBA, EdM, who is a dermatologist; and Jason Silverman, M.D., MSc., FRCPC, who is a pediatric gastroenterologist. I cannot thank you all enough for your candor and thoroughness, and also for all you do to help people every single day in so many ways–you are all the definition of heroes!

To my many (many!) sensitivity readers as well as the teachers, guidance counselors, students, scientists, parents, and other manuscript readers and photo reviewers . . . I'm forever grateful to you all for candidly sharing your varied perspectives and vulnerabilities with me to help me make this book as inclusive as possible.

Brynne Zaniboni, you are a gifted photographer that I am honored to work with. To my book models . . . my amazeballs book models . . . y'all are just priceless and incredible humans–thank you! Uttera Singh, you were so clutch during the production of this book and I am so grateful to you.

To my incredible manager Jane Startz: there are no words that can express how much I appreciate your kindness, brilliance, thoroughness, and positivity. I will never stop being grateful for all your nurturing, motivational, and positive encouragement throughout the years–I've learned so many life lessons from you, and not just about our industry. You are the ultimate role model. And to Jim Hornstein– you're just the cat's meow (even though y'all are dog parents!).

To all my wonderful extended family, friends, framily, mentors, and role models for the immense amount of support—there's no way I can thank everyone by name but the lengthy list includes Amanda (the best mommy in the world), Sammy (the best big brother in the world), Sunita and Jahar (the best in-laws a girl could have), Natasha, Charise, Natalie, Maya, Allison, Arianne, Lonye, Tanya, Julie Ann, Jinko, Mommy Jane, Kate, Tracy, Kalee, Cherise, Allegra, GayGay, Kaitlyn, Kiara, Nia, Lauren, Courtney, Caitlyn, Caira, Mary Beth, Kami . . . the list could go on and on, and the day this goes to print I'm sure I'll wake up in the middle of the night remembering the names of a few beloved people that I forgot to include in this list, and for that I'm sincerely apologetic in advance. But know that any omissions are simply accidental. As I tell my kids: nobody's perfect and everyone's doing their best!

Finally, thank you to my beloved hubby, Rupak, for always encouraging me and for loving me just as I am, and of course tremendous gratitude to our kiddos August and Nancy Rupali for not just inspiring this book but also being the most amazing people we could ask to have the honor of raising.

notes

Body Skin & Facial Skin

2 **Skin is the body's largest, heaviest:** "How Does Skin Work?," Institute for Quality and Efficiency in Health Care, last updated April 11, 2019, https://www.ncbi.nlm.nih .gov/books/NBK279255.

2 **15 percent of your body weight:** Isabella J. McLoughlin et al., "Skin Microbiome—the Next Frontier for Probiotic Intervention," *Probiotics and Antimicrobial Proteins* 14, no. 4 (2022): 630–47, https://doi.org /10.1007/s12602-021-09824-1.

2 **Shielding our bodies:** Fingani Annie Mphande, "The Structure and Function of the Skin," in *Skin Disorders in Vulnerable Populations: Causes, Impacts and Challenges* (Springer Singapore, 2020): 13–22.

2 **Producing hormones crucial to:** C. C. Zouboulis, "The Skin as an Endocrine Organ," *Dermato-Endocrinology* 1, no. 5 (September 2009): 250–52, https://doi .org/10.4161/derm.1.5.9499; Daniel D. Bikle, "Vitamin D and the Skin: Physiology and Pathophysiology," *Reviews in Endocrine and Metabolic Disorders* 13, no. 1 (August 2011): 3–19, https://doi.org/10.1007/s11154-011 -9194-0.

2 **Storing water, fat, and other products:** Mphande, "The Structure and Function of the Skin."

3 **The epidermis is the top skin layer:** Sarah de Szalay and Philip W. Wertz, "Protective Barriers Provided by the Epidermis," *International Journal of Molecular Sciences* 24, no. 4 (2023): 3145.

3 **melanin is produced:** "Layers of the Skin," National Cancer Institute SEER Training Modules accessed January 9, 2024, https://training.seer.cancer.gov /melanoma/anatomy/layers.html.

3 **renewing itself every twenty-eight days:** Adone Baroni et al., "Structure and Function of the Epidermis Related to Barrier Properties," *Clinics in Dermatology* 30, no. 3 (2012): 257–62.

3 **The dermis, the middle skin layer:** Juliet M. Pullar, Anitra C. Carr, and Margreet C. M. Vissers, "The Roles of Vitamin C in Skin Health," *Nutrients* 9, no. 8 (2017): 866; Bonnie D. Hodge, Terrence Sanvictores, and Robert T. Brodell, "Anatomy, Skin Sweat Glands," StatPearls, last updated October 10, 2022, https://www.ncbi.nlm .nih.gov/books/NBK482278; "Dermis," Cleveland Clinic, last updated February 7, 2022, https://my.clevelandclinic.org /health/body/22357-dermis.

3 **The bottom skin layer, the hypodermis:** "Hypodermis (Subcutaneous Tissue)," Cleveland Clinic, last updated October 19, 2021, https://my.clevelandclinic.org /health/body/21902-hypodermis -subcutaneous-tissue; Joyce Y. Kim and Harry Dao, "Physiology, Integument," StatPearls, last updated May 1, 2023, https://www.ncbi.nlm.nih.gov/books /NBK554386; Helen K. Graham et al., "Human Skin: Composition, Structure and Visualisation Methods," in *Skin Biophysics: From Experimental Characterisation to Advanced Modelling* (Springer, 2019), 1–18.

3 **Skin is thickest on:** Hani Yousef, Mandy Alhajj, and Sandeep Sharma, "Anatomy, Skin (Integument), Epidermis," StatPearls, last updated November 14, 2022, https:// www.ncbi.nlm.nih.gov/books/NBK470464.

3 **Facial skin is much thinner:** S. W. Lanigan and Zohra Zaidi, "Skin: Structure and Function," in *Dermatology in Clinical Practice* (Springer London, 2010): 1–15.

3 **most delicate skin is on the eyelids:** Miranda A. Farage, "Perceived Sensitive Skin at Different Anatomical Sites," in *Sensitive Skin Syndrome* 2nd ed., eds. Golara Honari, Rosa Andersen, and Howard L. Maibach (CRC Press, 2017), 117–35.

3 **Sweat is mostly water:** Lindsay B. Baker, "Physiology of Sweat Gland Function: The Roles of Sweating and Sweat Composition in Human Health," *Temperature* 6, no. 3 (2019): 211–59, https://doi.org10.1080/23328940.2019.1632145.

3 **sweat exits the body:** Baker, "Physiology of Sweat Gland Function."

4 **Humans have millions:** Andy Blow, "Why Do Humans Sweat So Much?," Precision Fuel & Hydration, accessed January 9, 2024 https://www.precisionhydration.com/performance-advice/hydration/why-do-humans-sweat-so-much.

4 **This unusual capacity enables us:** Hodge, Sanvictores, and Brodell, "Anatomy, Skin Sweat Glands."

4 **Some people sweat more intensely:** Jan Havlíček, Jitka Fialová, and S. Craig Roberts, "Individual Variation in Body Odor," in *Springer Handbook of Odor* (Springer, 2017): 125–26.

4 **hyperhidrosis, which is the medical term:** Jason E. Sammons and Amor Khachemoune, "Axillary Hyperhidrosis: A Focused Review," *Journal of Dermatological Treatment* 28, no. 7 (2017): 582–90, https://doi.org/10.1080/09546634.2017.1309347.

4 **make you feel uncomfortable:** Kristeen Cherney. "Anxiety Got You in a Sweat? Why Anxiety Sweating Happens and How to Handle It," Healthline, last updated May 31, 2023, https://www.healthline.com/health/diagnosing-hyperhidrosis/depression-and-anxiety.

4 **This condition is called hypohidrosis:** Melissa Mei Hsia Chan et al., "Isolated Hypohidrosis: Pathogenesis and Treatment," *European Journal of Dermatology* 30, no. 6 (2020): 680–87, https://doi.org/10.1684/ejd.2020.3931.

4 **ability to sweat decreasing:** Charlotte Lillis, "What to Know about Hypohidrosis," MedicalNewsToday, last updated July 20, 2023, https://www.medicalnewstoday.com/articles/322193.

4 **rare but harmless condition called chromhidrosis:** Dustin Wilkes and Shivaraj Nagalli, "Chromhidrosis," StatPearls, last updated July 3, 2023, https://pubmed.ncbi.nlm.nih.gov/32119282/.

5 **too long, odor arises:** Havlíček, Fialová, and Roberts, "Individual Variation in Body Odor."

5 **Most sweat glands are eccrine glands:** Britta De Pessemier et al., "Underarm Body Odor, the Microbiome, and Probiotic Treatment," in *Good Microbes in Medicine, Food Production, Biotechnology, Bioremediation, and Agriculture* (Wiley, 2022): 52–63.

5 **Apocrine glands produce a thicker type:** Valentina Parma et al., "Processing of Human Body Odors," in *Springer Handbook of Odor*, 127–28.

5 **aren't activated until puberty:** Chris Callewaert, Jo Lambert, and Tom Van de Wiele, "Towards a Bacterial Treatment for Armpit Malodour," *Experimental Dermatology* 26, no. 5 (2017): 388–91, https://doi.org/10.1111/exd.13259.

5 **count as pheromones:** Bhupendra C. Patel et al., "Anatomy, Skin, Sudoriferous Gland," StatPearls, last updated April 24, 2023,

https://www.ncbi.nlm.nih.gov/books /NBK513244.

5 **sweat and dirt stay on your skin:** "Body Odor: Causes, Changes, Underlying Diseases and Treatment," Cleveland Clinic, last updated March 4, 2022, https:// my.clevelandclinic.org/health/symptoms /17865-body-odor.

5 **Bathing with soap and water:** "Sweating and Body Odor," Mayo Clinic, October 27, 2021, https://www.mayoclinic.org /diseases-conditions/sweating-and-body -odor/diagnosis-treatment/drc-20353898.

6 **without washing between wears:** Charlotte Hilton Andersen, "Here's What Happens If You Don't Change Your Underwear," The Healthy, last updated September 11, 2023, https://www.thehealthy.com/habits/heres -what-happens-if-you-dont-change-your -underwear.

6 **Polyester, rayon, and nylon:** Mohammed M. Abdul-Bari et al., "Synthetic Clothing and the Problem with Odor: Comparison of Nylon and Polyester Fabrics," *Clothing and Textiles Research Journal* 36, no. 4 (2018): 251–66, https://doi.org/10.1177 /0887302X18772099.

6 **such as cotton or linen:** Andreas Møllebjerg et al., "The Bacterial Life Cycle in Textiles Is Governed by Fiber Hydrophobicity," *Microbiology Spectrum* 9, no. 2 (2021): e01185–21, https://doi.org/10.1128 /Spectrum.01185-21.

6 **the aroma of pungent foods:** James A. Peterson, "Shareable Resource: Ten Things to Know about Body Odor," *ACSM's Health and Fitness Journal* 22, no. 3 (2018): 48, https://doi.org10.1249/FIT .0000000000000393.

6 **People who are sick or very stressed:** Pearlin Shabna Naziz, Runima Das, and Supriyo Sen, "The Scent of Stress: Evidence from the Unique Fragrance of

Agarwood," *Frontiers in Plant Science* 10 (2019): 840, https://doi.org/10.3389 /fpls.2019.00840.

6 **a medical condition called bromhidrosis:** Ali S. Malik, Caroline L. Porter, and Steven R. Feldman, "Bromhidrosis Treatment Modalities: A Literature Review," *Journal of the American Academy of Dermatology* 89, no. 1 (2021): 81–89, https://doi.org /10.1016/j.jaad.2021.01.030.

6 **which means "foul-smelling sweat":** "Bromhidrosis," in *Merriam-Webster Dictionary*, accessed January 9, 2024, https://www.merriam-webster.com /medical/bromhidrosis.

6 **bacteria on their bodies:** Malik, Porter, and Feldman, "Bromhidrosis Treatment Modalities."

6 **"old person smell":** Kimberly Holland, "Do Older People Actually Smell Different?," Healthline, October 25, 2018, https://www .healthline.com/health/older-people-smell -different#treatment.

7 **a reputation for reducing odor:** Matthew Elliott, "Eat the Right Foods to Say Goodbye to Body Odor," *LifeHack*, last updated January 2, 2017, https://www .lifehack.org/506004/eat-the-right-foods -to-say-goodbye-to-body-odor.

7 **known to cause "maple syrup sweat":** Upma Singh et al., "Amazing Health Benefit of Fenugreek," *International Journal of Environment and Health Sciences* 4, no. 2 (2022): 19–27, https://doi.org/10.47062 /1190.0402.03.

7 **trimming or removing body fuzz:** Zoe Diana Draelos, "Cosmeceuticals for Male Skin," *Dermatologic Clinics* 36, no. 1 (2018): 17–20.

7 **Antiperspirants block sweat glands:** Eric S. Abrutyn, "Antiperspirants and Deodorants," in *Cosmetic Dermatology:*

Products and Procedures (Wiley, 2022), 213–22.

7 **deodorants don't stop you from sweating:** Erika CV de Oliveira et al., "Deodorants and Antiperspirants: Identification of New Strategies and Perspectives to Prevent and Control Malodor and Sweat of the Body," *International Journal of Dermatology* 60, no. 5 (2021): 613–19, https://doi.org/10.1111/ijd.15418.

7 **all-in-one combination or separately:** Amina Bouslimani et al., "The Impact of Skin Care Products on Skin Chemistry and Microbiome Dynamics," *BMC Biology* 17 (2019): 1–20.

7 **Products marked "clinical":** Rachael Schultz, "The 15 Best Clinical Strength Deodorants and Antiperspirants of 2023, Tested and Reviewed," Verywell Health, March 16, 2023, https://www.verywell health.com/best-clinical-strength -deodorants-4687662.

8 **prescription options available:** Gulhima Arora et al., "Treatment of Axillary Hyperhidrosis," *Journal of Cosmetic Dermatology* 21, no. 1 (2022): 62–70, https://doi.org/10.1111/jocd.14378.

8 **symptoms of a medical condition:** Adam Felman, "What to Know about Body Odor," MedicalNewsToday, last updated April 24, 2023, https://www.medicalnewstoday .com/articles/173478.

8 **might be offensive:** Caroline Tang, "Why One Person's Sweet Scent Is Another's Foul Odour," UNSW Sydney, June 23, 2020, https://newsroom.unsw.edu.au /news/science-tech/why-one-person %E2%80%99s-sweet-scent-another %E2%80%99s-foul-odour.

8 **bacteria called brevibacterium:** Nobuhiro Asai et al., "*Brevibacterium paucivorans* Bacteremia: Case Report and Review of the Literature," *BMC Infectious Diseases* 19,

no. 1 (2019): 344, https://doi.org/10.1186 /s12879-019-3962-y.

8 **bacteria used to produce:** Morgan Petruny, "Stinking Up the Test Zone," *Runner's World* 55, no. 2 (2020): 82–83.

8 **Are your feet bringing the funk?:** Karen Asp, "Tips for Healthy Feet," WebMD, June 11, 2015, https://www.webmd.com /skin-problems-and-treatments/healthy -feet-tips.

8 **"toe jam," which develops when:** "What Is Toe Jam?," UPMC HealthBeat, March 29, 2022, https://share.upmc.com/2015/10 /how-to-prevent-toe-jam.

9 **Dry feet have less chance:** Felman, "What to Know about Body Odor."

9 **like athlete's foot:** "Athlete's Foot (Tinea Pedis)," Cleveland Clinic, last updated December 1, 2021, https:// my.clevelandclinic.org/health/diseases /22139-athletes-foot-tinea-pedis.

9 **tips to prevent:** Asp, "Tips for Healthy Feet."

11 **between 5 and 10 percent of Americans:** W. Erickson, C. Lee, and S. von Schrader, *2018 Disability Status Report: United States* (Cornell University Yang-Tan Institute on Employment and Disability, 2018).

15 **known as lipids:** Anastasia P. Nesterova et al., "Diseases of the Skin and Subcutaneous Tissue," in *Disease Pathways: An Atlas of Human Disease Signaling Pathways* (Elsevier, 2019), 493–532, https://doi.org/10.1016/b978-0 -12-817086-1.00011-7.

15 **scratching can easily damage:** Catharina Sagita Moniaga, Mitsutoshi Tominaga, and Kenji Takamori, "Mechanisms and Management of Itch in Dry Skin," *Acta Dermato-Venereologica* 100, no. 2 (2020): 9–20, https://doi.org/10.2340 /00015555-3344.

15 techniques to help keep: "Skin Care: 5 Tips for Healthy Skin," Mayo Clinic, January 22, 2022, https://www.mayoclinic.org/healthy -lifestyle/adult-health/in-depth/skin-care /art-20048237.

15 buildup of dead skin cells: Matthias Augustin et al., "Diagnosis and Treatment of Xerosis Cutis—A Position Paper," *Journal der Deutschen Dermatologischen Gesellschaft* 17, no. S7 (2019): 3–33, https://doi.org/10.1111/ddg.13906.

15 stimulates new skin cell growth: Whitney Bowe, *Dirty Looks: The Secret to Beautiful Skin* (Little, Brown Spark, 2019).

16 coconut oil can be a good choice: Shashank Joshi et al., "Coconut Oil and Immunity: What Do We Really Know about It So Far?," *Journal of the Association of Physicians of India* 68, no. 7 (2020): 67–72, https:// pubmed.ncbi.nlm.nih.gov/32602684/.

16 extremely dry skin is "xerosis": Augustin, et al., "Diagnosis and Treatment of Xerosis Cutis."

17 Lips help us eat, speak: Meghan A. Piccinin and Patrick M. Zito, "Anatomy, Head and Neck, Lips," StatPearls, last updated June 5, 2023, https://pubmed .ncbi.nlm.nih.gov/29939677/.

17 And your lip imprint: Amita Negi and Anurag Negi, "The Connecting Link! Lip Prints and Fingerprints," *Journal of Forensic Dental Sciences* 8, no. 3 (2016): 177, https://www.ncbi.nlm.nih.gov/pmc /articles/PMC5210114.

17 easy ways to heal chapped lips: "7 Dermatologists' Tips for Healing Dry, Chapped Lips," American Academy of Dermatology Association accessed January 4, 2024, https://www.aad.org /public/everyday-care/skin-care-basics /dry/heal-dry-chapped-lips.

17 a condition like angular cheilitis: Justin R. Federico, Brandon M. Basehore, and Patrick M. Zito, "Angular Chelitis," StatPearls, last updated March 7, 2023, https://www.statpearls.com/point-of -care/32719.

17 most people have HSV: Kimberly Velarde, "Herpes Simplex Virus 1 Amplicon Vectors," PhD diss., Arizona State University, 2021.

18 a cold sore or fever blister: "Fever Blisters and Canker Sores," National Institute of Dental and Craniofacial Research, last updated September 2021, https://www .nidcr.nih.gov/health-info/fever-blisters -canker-sores; "Cold Sores," Cleveland Clinic, last updated April 27, 2023, https:// my.clevelandclinic.org/health/diseases /21136-cold-sores.

18 sore on your sexual partner: "How Is Herpes Prevented?," Planned Parenthood accessed January 4, 2024, https://www .plannedparenthood.org/learn/stds-hiv -safer-sex/herpes/how-is-herpes-prevented.

19 clogged by oil, sweat: "Acne," Johns Hopkins Medicine, accessed January 9, 2024, https://www.hopkinsmedicine.org /health/conditions-and-diseases/acne.

19 4 out of every 5: Darren Lynn et al., "The Epidemiology of Acne Vulgaris in Late Adolescence," *Adolescent Health, Medicine and Therapeutics* 7 (2015): 7–13, https:// doi.org/10.2147/ahmt.s55832.

19 different types of acne: "Acne," National Institute of Arthritis and Musculoskeletal and Skin Diseases, last updated July 2023, https://www.niams.nih.gov/health-topics /acne; Debra Fulghum Bruce, "Teens and Acne," WebMD, last updated February 10, 2023, https:// www.webmd.com/skin-problems-and -treatments/acne/what-is-acne.

20 cysts, which are sacs: "Cysts (Overview)," Harvard Health, March 9, 2022, https:// www.health.harvard.edu/a_to_z/cysts -overview-a-to-z.

20 **more pimple-causing bacteria:** Dylan Alston, "Should You Pop That Pimple?," Intermountainhealthcare.org (blog), April 17, 2019, https://intermountainhealthcare.org/blogs/should-you-pop-that-pimple.

21 **late teens or early twenties:** "Acne in Adolescents and Young Adults," Johns Hopkins Medicine, December 13, 2021, https://www.hopkinsallchildrens.org/ACH-News/General-News/Acne-in-Adolescents-and-Young-Adults.

22 **dirty, bacteria-covered material:** Rachel Lapidos, "Forehead Breaking Out? The Surprising Reason Your Hat Could Be to Blame," *Well+Good*, May 13, 2019, https://www.wellandgood.com/forehead-breakout.

22 **Stress makes acne worse:** Diana Wells, "The Relationship between Stress and Acne," Healthline, August 14, 2018, https://www.healthline.com/health/stress-acne.

23 **has a skin-picking disorder:** Jeanne Fama, "What Is Skin Picking Disorder?," International OCD Foundation, accessed January 9, 2024, https://iocdf.org/about-ocd/related-disorders/skin-picking-disorder.

23 **severe pain and scarring:** Jon E. Grant and Samuel R. Chamberlain, "Trichotillomania and Skin-Picking Disorder: An Update," *Focus* 19, no. 4 (2021): 405–12, https://doi.org/10.1176/appi.focus.20210013.

23 **disorder, called dermatillomania:** Stephania L. Hayes, Eric A. Storch, and Lissette Berlanga, "Skin Picking Behaviors: An Examination of the Prevalence and Severity in a Community Sample," *Journal of Anxiety Disorders* 23, no. 3 (2009): 314–19, https://doi.org/10.1016/j.janxdis.2009.01.008.

23 **also have trichotillomania:** Jon E. Grant and Samuel R. Chamberlain, "Characteristics of 262 Adults with Skin Picking Disorder," *Comprehensive Psychiatry* 117 (2022): 152338, https://doi.org/10.1016/j.comppsych.2022.152338.

23 **follicles are found almost everywhere:** Heather L. Brannon, "Sebaceous Glands and Your Skin," Verywell Health, last updated July 1, 2022, https://www.verywellhealth.com/sebaceous-glands-1069374.

24 **types of folliculitis:** Margaret W. Mann and Daniel L. Popkin, eds., *Handbook of Dermatology: A Practical Manual* (Wiley, 2019).

25 **called a carbuncle:** "Boils and Carbuncles," Cleveland Clinic, last updated October 11, 2021, https://my.clevelandclinic.org/health/diseases/15153-boils-and-carbuncles.

25 **folliculitis will go away by itself:** James Roland, "Folliculitis: What It Is and What You Can Do about It," Healthline, last updated February 9, 2023, https://www.healthline.com/health/folliculitis.

25 **the goose bumps disappear:** Sharon Reynolds, "What Goosebumps Are For," National Institutes of Health, July 28, 2020, https://www.nih.gov/news-events/nih-research-matters/what-goosebumps-are.

26 **born with the freckle gene:** "MC1R Gene," MedlinePlus, https://medlineplus.gov/genetics/gene/mc1r; Beth Sissons, "What to Know about Freckles," MedicalNewsToday, October 26, 2018, https://www.medicalnewstoday.com/articles/323471#causes; "Freckles (Ephelides and Solar Lentigines)," Cleveland Clinic, last updated May 23, 2022, https://my.clevelandclinic.org/health/articles/23091-freckles.

26 **Warts are rough-surfaced:** Elea Carey, "Everything You Need to Know about Warts," Healthline, last updated February 14, 2023, https://www.healthline.com/health/skin/warts.

26 **Warts are very contagious:** "Warts: Overview," InformedHealth.org, last updated November 7, 2019, https://www .ncbi.nlm.nih.gov/books/NBK279586/.

26 **Most warts disappear:** "Warts," Cedars-Sinai, accessed January 9, 2024, https:// www.cedars-sinai.org/health-library /diseases-and-conditions/w/warts.html.

26 **plantar (foot) warts:** "Plantar Warts," Mayo Clinic, last updated March 29, 2023, https://www.mayoclinic.org/diseases -conditions/plantar-warts/symptoms -causes/syc-20352691.

27 **virus is easily transmitted:** "Molluscum Contagiosum," Centers for Disease Control and Prevention, last updated May 11, 2015, https://www.cdc.gov/poxvirus/molluscum -contagiosum/index.html.

27 **They aren't contagious:** Yvette Brazier, "All You Need to Know about Skin Tags," MedicalNewsToday, last updated April 17, 2023, https://www.medicalnewstoday .com/articles/67317.

27 **grow extra cells:** Brazier, "All You Need to Know about Skin Tags."

27 **risk of extreme bleeding and infection:** Cory Martin, "How to Remove a Skin Tag," Health, March 10, 2023, https://www .health.com/skin-tag-removal-7111825.

27 **Some moles are hereditary:** "Moles: What They Are, Causes, Types and Examination," Cleveland Clinic, last updated February 2, 2021, https://my.clevelandclinic.org /health/diseases/4410-moles; "Common Moles, Dysplastic Nevi, and Risk of Melanoma," National Cancer Institute, last updated November 17, 2022, https://www .cancer.gov/types/skin/moles-fact-sheet.

28 **moles should be closely monitored:** Melanie Dixon, "The ABCDEs of Moles," Mayo Clinic Health System, April. 4, 2022, https://www.mayoclinichealthsystem.org /hometown-health/speaking-of-health /the-abcdes-of-moles.

28 **skin cancer detection ABCDEs:** Dixon, "The ABCDEs of Moles."

29 **taking pictures every:** Amanda Capritto, "4 Ways to Spot Skin Cancer with Your Smartphone," CNET, June 27, 2023, https://www.cnet.com/health/personal -care/how-to-use-your-smartphone-to -detect-skin-cancer/.

29 **like wrinkle prevention:** Vivien Lai, William Cranwell, and Rodney Sinclair, "Epidemiology of Skin Cancer in the Mature Patient," *Clinics in Dermatology* 36, no. 2 (2018): 167–76, https://doi.org/10.1016/j .clindermatol.2017.10.008.

29 **Dark Skin Needs Skin Cancer Screenings:** Ak Gupta, Mausumi Bharadwaj, and Ravi Mehrotra, "Skin Cancer Concerns in People of Color: Risk Factors and Prevention," *Asian Pacific Journal of Cancer Prevention* 17, no. 12: 5257–64, https://doi .org/10.22034/apjcp.2016.17.12.5257.

29 **skin cancers caused by UV rays:** "Skin Cancer in People of Color," Columbia University Irving Medical Center, May 3, 2022, https://www.cuimc.columbia.edu /news/skin-cancer-people-color.

29 **several moles, close relatives:** "Melanoma," Mayo Clinic, last updated July 22, 2023, https://www.mayoclinic.org/diseases -conditions/melanoma/symptoms-causes /syc-20374884.

29 **anyone can be diagnosed:** "Is Sun Exposure the Only Cause of Skin Cancer?," UPMC Western Maryland, March 20, 2018, https://www.wmhs.com/sun-exposure -cause-skin-cancer/.

29 **best avoid carcinogenic:** "Sun Safety," Centers for Disease Control and Prevention, last updated April 18, 2023, https://www.cdc.gov/cancer/skin/basic _info/sun-safety.htm.

30 **at least 30 SPF:** Loren E. Hernandez et al., "Sunscreen Compliance with American Academy of Dermatology Recommendations: A 2022 Update and Cross-Sectional Study," *Journal of the American Academy of Dermatology* 88, no. 1 (2023): 231–32, https://doi.org/10.1016/j.jaad.2022.05.003.

30 **prevention of some types of skin cancer:** Emilia Kanasuo et al., "Regular Use of Vitamin D Supplement Is Associated with Fewer Melanoma Cases Compared to Non-Use: A Cross-Sectional Study in 498 Adult Subjects at Risk of Skin Cancers," *Melanoma Research* 33, no. 2 (2023): 126–35, https://doi.org/10.1097/CMR-0000000000000870.

31 **skin cancers on the hand:** Colleen Moriarty, "Q&A: What to Know before Heading to a Nail Salon," Yale Medicine, July 28, 2023, https://www.yalemedicine.org/news/what-to-know-before-heading-to-a-nail-salon.

31 **Cellulite isn't considered a medical:** "Cellulite," Cleveland Clinic, last updated October 28, 2021, https://my.clevelandclinic.org/health/diseases/17694-cellulite.

31 **10 percent of people:** "Cellulite," Cleveland Clinic.

32 **cardiovascular work tightens:** Katey Davidson, "Is It Possible to Get Rid of Cellulite with Exercises?," Healthline, last updated April 27, 2022, https://www.healthline.com/health/fitness-exercise/cellulite-exercises.

32 **scars we call stretch marks:** Ashley Marcin, "7 Tips to Help Prevent Stretch Marks," Healthline, last updated July 21, 2023, https://www.healthline.com/health/how-to-prevent-stretch-marks.

32 **show up most:** Marcin, "7 Tips."

32 **history of stretch marks:** Marcin, "7 Tips."

33 **First, blood rushes to the injury:** "How Wounds Heal," Health Encyclopedia, University of Rochester Medical Center, accessed January 9, 2024, https://www.urmc.rochester.edu/encyclopedia/content.aspx?ContentTypeID=134&ContentID=143.

33 **injuries leave scars:** "Scars: Treatment and Cause," Cleveland Clinic, last updated March 15, 2021, https://my.clevelandclinic.org/health/diseases/11030-scars.

33 **Superficial scars, meaning:** "Scars," Cleveland Clinic.

33 **are more obvious:** "Scars and Your Skin," WebMD, last updated January 18, 2022, https://www.webmd.com/skin-problems-and-treatments/scars.

33 **prevent infection and scarring:** "Proper Wound Care: How to Minimize a Scar," American Academy of Dermatology Association, accessed January 9, 2024, https://www.aad.org/public/everyday-care/injured-skin/burns/wound-care-minimize-scars.

34 **puckered tissue called keloids:** Brian Berman, Andrea Maderal, and Brian Raphael, "Keloids and Hypertrophic Scars: Pathophysiology, Classification, and Treatment," *Dermatologic Surgery* 43, suppl. 1 (2017): S3–S18.

34 **medication to help stave off:** Udayan Betarbet and Travis W. Blalock, "Keloids: A Review of Etiology, Prevention, and Treatment," *Journal of Clinical and Aesthetic Dermatology* 13, no. 2 (2020): 33–43, https://www.ncbi.nlm.nih.gov/pmc/articles/PMC7158916.

34 **to fully heal:** Karishma Daftary and Walter Liszewski, "Tattoo-Related Allergic Contact Dermatitis," *Current Dermatology Reports* 11, no. 4 (2022): 202–8.

35 **avoiding piercing guns:** "Issues with Piercing Guns," Association of Professional

Piercers, accessed January 9, 2024, https://safepiercing.org/piercing-guns.

35 impossible to fully sterilize: "Body Piercings, Teens and Potential Health Risks: AAP Report Explained," Healthy Children, last updated April 28, 2021, https://www.healthychildren.org/English /ages-stages/teen/Pages/body-piercings .aspx.

35 nerve damage is possible: "What to Know about Oral Piercing," WebMD, January 24, 2023, https://www.webmd.com/oral -health/oral-piercing; Valencia Higuera, "Getting Tattooed or Pierced," Healthline, last updated August 31, 2020, https:// www.healthline.com/health/beauty-skin -care-tattoos-piercings.

35 impossible—to remove: Wan Chee Kwang, "3 Big Reasons Why Your Tattoo Could Be Impossible to Remove," 1Aesthetics, Medical & Surgery, December 10, 2022, https://1aesthetics.com/3-big-reasons -why-your-tattoo-could-be-impossible-to -remove/.

35 Signs your tattoo or piercing might be infected: Susan Massick, "How to Prevent a Tattoo Infection," Ohio State Health and Discovery, July 25, 2022, https://health .osu.edu/health/virus-and-infection/how -to-prevent-a-tattoo-infection.

36 compromise condom use: Dayton Preslar and Judith Borger, "Body Piercing Infections," StatPearls, last updated July 10, 2023, https://www.ncbi.nlm.nih .gov/books/NBK537336/.

36 Mouth piercings can: Nicole Müller et al., "'Body Modification: Piercing and Tattooing in Congenital Heart Disease Patients,' Decoration or Disaster? A Narrative Review," *Cardiovascular Diagnosis and Therapy* 11, no. 6 (2021): 1395–402, https://doi.org/10.21037/cdt-21-458.

36 piercing might stretch: India Bottomley, "How to Fix Old and Sagging Piercings," The Aedition, February 7, 2019, https://aedit .com/aedition/how-to-fix-old-and-sagging -piercings.

37 Vitiligo. Millions of people: Kavita Gandhi et al., "Prevalence of Vitiligo among Adults in the United States," *JAMA Dermatology* 158, no. 1 (2022): 43–50; https://doi.org /10.1001/jamadermatol.2021.4724.

37 Vitiligo often begins: Paula Ludmann, "Vitiligo: Causes," American Academy of Dermatology Association, last updated June 29, 2022, https://www.aad.org /public/diseases/a-z/vitiligo-causes.

37 there are treatments available: Michelle Rodrigues et al., "Current and Emerging Treatments for Vitiligo," *Journal of the American Academy of Dermatology* 77, no. 1 (2017): 17–29, https://doi.org /10.1016/j.jaas.2016.11.010.

37 no or very little melanin: "Albinism: Types, Symptoms and Causes," Cleveland Clinic, last updated August 5, 2021, https://my .clevelandclinic.org/health/diseases/21747 -albinism.

38 When melanocytes are: "Melanin: What Is It, Types and Benefits," Cleveland Clinic, last updated March 29, 2022, https:// my.clevelandclinic.org/health/body/22615 -melanin.

38 body's coloration is genetic: Romain Madelaine et al., "Genetic Deciphering of the Antagonistic Activities of the Melanin-Concentrating Hormone and Melanocortin Pathways in Skin Pigmentation," *PLoS Genetics* 16, no.12 (2020): e1009244, https://doi.org/10.1371/journal.pgen .1009244.

38 screening for certain medical conditions: Mohammad Abid Keen, Iffat Hassan Shah, and Gousia Sheikh, "Cutaneous Manifestations of Polycystic Ovary

Syndrome: A Cross-Sectional Clinical Study," *Indian Dermatology Online Journal* 8, no. 2 (2017): 104–10, https://doi.org/10.4103/2229-5178.202275; Angelina Labib, Jordan Rosen, and Gil Yosipovitch, "Skin Manifestations of Diabetes Mellitus," in *Endotext,* eds. Angelina Labib, Jordan Rosen, and Gil Yosipovitch (MDText.com, Inc., 2022), https://www.ncbi.nlm.nih.gov/books/NBK481900.

38 **Sun exposure. UV rays:** K. A. Merin, Merin Shaji, and R. Kameswaran, "A Review on Sun Exposure and Skin Diseases," *Indian Journal of Dermatology* 67, no. 5 (2022): 625, https://doi.org/10.4103/ijd.ijd_1092_20.

38 **Friction and movement:** MaryAnn De Pietro, "What You Should Know about Hyperpigmentation," Healthline, last updated September 11, 2023, https://www.healthline.com/health/hyperpigmentation.

38 **Skin damage. Razor burn:** "Hyperpigmentation: Age Spots, Sun Spots, and Liver Spots," Cleveland Clinic, last updated October 7, 2021, https://my.clevelandclinic.org/health/diseases/21885-hyperpigmentation.

39 **heavily lotion the darker spots:** Hawasatu Dumbuya et al., "Efficacy of Ceramide-Containing Formulations on UV-Induced Skin Surface Barrier Alterations," *Journal of Drugs in Dermatology* 20, no. 4 (2021): S29–S35, https://doi.org/10.36849/JDD.2021.589E.

39 **darken after puberty:** Simone Scully, "Read This If You're Asking Yourself, 'Why Is My Private Area Dark?,'" Healthline, February 11, 2021, https://www.healthline.com/health/why-is-my-private-area-dark#triggers-to-avoid.

40 **eczema, psoriasis, and rosacea:** Rosalyn Carson-DeWitt, "Psoriasis vs. Eczema vs. Rosacea: What's the Difference?," Verywell Health, last updated November 1, 2022, https://www.verywellhealth.com/do-you-have-rosacea-psoriasis-or-eczema-3892103.

41 **Similar to atopic dermatitis:** Yan Li and Linfeng Li, "Contact Dermatitis: Classifications and Management," *Clinical Reviews in Allergy and Immunology* 61, no. 3 (2021): 245–81, https://doi.org/0.1007/s12016-021-08875-0.

41 **Triggered by prescribed:** "Drug Rashes," Johns Hopkins Medicine, November 19, 2019, https://www.hopkinsmedicine.org/health/conditions-and-diseases/drug-rashes.

42 **a chafing rash:** "Chafing: Causes and Prevention," Cleveland Clinic, last updated July 19, 2022, https://my.clevelandclinic.org/health/diseases/23517-chafing.

42 **skin condition called intertrigo:** Timothy Nobles and Richard A. Miller, "Intertrigo," StatPearls, last updated September 19, 2022, https://www.ncbi.nlm.nih.gov/books/NBK531489/.

42 **found in the armpit:** Ahmet Metin, Nursel Dilek, and Serap Gunes Bilgili, "Recurrent Candidal Intertrigo: Challenges and Solutions," *Clinical, Cosmetic and Investigational Dermatology* 11 (2018): 175–85, https://doi.org/10.2147CCID.S127841.

42 **an annoying rash:** "Fungal Diseases," National Institute of Allergy and Infectious Diseases, last updated October 26, 2018, https://www.niaid.nih.gov/diseases-conditions/fungal-diseases.

42 **It's called ringworm:** "About Ringworm," Centers for Disease Control and Prevention, last updated February 26, 2021, https://www.cdc.gov/fungal/diseases/ringworm/definition.html.

43 **and/or clumpy discharge:** "*Candida auris*," Centers for Disease Control and Prevention, last updated September 26,

2023, https://www.cdc.gov/fungal/candida-auris/index.html.

44 **keep foot fungus:** Heather Grey, "Everything You Need to Know about Fungal Infection," Healthline, last updated March 8, 2019, https://www.healthline.com/health/fungal-infection.

44 **for fungal infections:** "Fungal Nail Infections," Centers for Disease Control and Prevention, last updated September 13, 2022, https://www.cdc.gov/fungal/nail-infections.html.

44 **known as onychomycosis:** "Fungal Nail Infections," Centers for Disease Control and Prevention.

44 **get the right medication:** "Nail Fungus: Who Gets and Causes," American Academy of Dermatology Association accessed January 9, 2024, https://www.aad.org/public/diseases/a-z/nail-fungus-causes.

44 **among people of color:** Rosalind J. Mole and Duncan N. MacKenzie, "Subungual Melanoma," StatPearls, last updated April 14, 2023, https://www.ncbi.nlm.nih.gov/books/NBK482480/.

44 **is "skin appendage":** "Structure of the Nails," InformedHealth.org, June 28, 2018,https://www.ncbi.nlm.nih.gov/books/NBK513133/.

45 **improperly grow into the skin:** Eckart Haneke, "Controversies in the Treatment of Ingrown Nails," *Dermatology Research and Practice* 2012 (2012): 783924, https://doi.org/10.1155/2012/783924.

45 **soak your hand or foot:** "Ingrown Toenails," Mayo Clinic, February 8, 2022, https://www.mayoclinic.org/diseases-conditions/ingrown-toenails/diagnosis-treatment/drc-20355908.

46 **until the nail begins growing:** "Ingrown Toenails," Mayo Clinic.

46 **serious and permanent damage:** Shannon Johnson, "Ingrown Toenails: Why Do They Happen?," Healthline, last updated May 31, 2023, https://www.healthline.com/health/ingrown-toenail#complications.

46 **Up to 30 percent:** "How Biting Your Nails Is Affecting Your Health," UCLA Health, September 22, 2022, https://www.uclahealth.org/news/how-biting-your-nails-is-affecting-your-health.

46 **known as onychophagia:** Pierre Halteh, Richard K. Scher, and Shari R. Lipner, "Onychophagia: A Nail-Biting Conundrum for Physicians," *Journal of Dermatological Treatment* 28, no. 2 (2017): 166–72, https://doi.org/10.1080/09546634.2016.1200711.

46 **thickened areas of dead skin:** "Corns and Calluses," Mount Sinai Health System accessed January 9, 2024, org/health-library/diseases-conditions/corns-and-calluses.

46 **Calluses. Painless patches:** "Corns and Calluses," Mount Sinai Health System.

47 **by buffing them away:** Cheryl Whitten, "What Is a Pumice Stone?," WebMD, November 22, 2022, https://www.webmd.com/beauty/what-is-pumice-stone.

47 **smaller than calluses:** "Corns and Calluses," Mount Sinai Health System.

47 **difficult to remove:** "Corns: Overview," InformedHealth.org, April 11, 2019, https://www.ncbi.nlm.nih.gov/books/NBK541153/.

47 **Painful foot bumps:** "Bunions," OrthoInfo, American Academy of Orthopaedic Surgeons, last updated March 2022, https://orthoinfo.aaos.org/en/diseases—conditions/bunions.

48 **Millions of people become infested:** Nonye Ogbuefi and Brandi Kenner-Bell, "Common Pediatric Infestations: Update on Diagnosis and Treatment of Scabies, Head Lice, and Bed Bugs," *Current Opinion in*

Pediatrics 33, no. 4 (2021): 410–15, https://doi.org10.1097/MOP.0000000000001031.

48 **itchy, bumpy rashes:** Jim Powers and Talel Badri, "Pediculosis Corporis," StatPearls, last updated June 12, 2023, https://www.ncbi.nlm.nih.gov/books/NBK482148/.

48 **lice are contagious:** Elaine Webber and Sherry McConnell, "Lice Update: Management and Treatment in the Home," *Home Healthcare Now* 36, no. 5 (2018): 289–94, https://doi.org10.1097/NHH.0000000000000677.

48 **spread either of these:** P. U. Patel, A. Tan, and N. J. Levell, "A Clinical Review and History of Pubic Lice," *Clinical and Experimental Dermatology* 46, no. 7 (2021): 1181–88, https://doi.org10.1111/ced.14666.

48 **lice can transmit some illnesses:** Nadia Amanzougaghene et al., "Where Are We with Human Lice? A Review of the Current State of Knowledge," *Frontiers in Cellular and Infection Microbiology* 9 (2020): 474, https://doi.org/10.3389/fcimb.2019.00474.

48 **Scabies mites are:** "Scabies Frequently Asked Questions (FAQs)," Centers for Disease Control and Prevention, last updated September 1, 2020, https://www.cdc.gov/parasites/scabies/gen_info/faqs.html.

49 **body, head, and pubic lice:** Saied Reza Naddaf, "Lice, Humans, and Microbes," *Iranian Biomedical Journal* 22, no. 5 (2018): 292–3, https://www.ncbi.nlm.nih.gov/pmc/articles/PMC6058184.

49 **live in clothing and bedding:** "Parasites—Lice," Centers for Disease Control and Prevention, last updated September 11, 2019, https://www.cdc.gov/parasites/lice/.

49 **anywhere that hair grows:** Amanzougaghene et al., "Where Are We with Human Lice?"

49 **scabies or lice:** "Scabies Frequently Asked Questions (FAQs)," Centers for Disease Control and Prevention.

49 **to avoid reinfestation:** Annie Imboden, "Effective Treatments for Head Lice," *Nurse Practitioner* 44, no. 9 (2019): 36–42, https://doi.org10.1097/01.NPR.0000574668.19239.db.

49 **lice can't survive:** "Head Lice and Nits," NHS Inform, last updated January 18, 2023, https://www.nhsinform.scot/illnesses-and-conditions/skin-hair-and-nails/head-lice-and-nits.

50 **three main ways:** "Head Lice: Prevention and Control," Centers for Disease Control and Prevention, last updated September 12, 2019, https://www.cdc.gov/parasites/lice/head/prevent.html.

50 **eliminate lice eggs:** Sandra Raju et al., "Over the Counter: Head Lice," *Australian Pharmacist* 41, no. 4 (2022): 44–52.

50 **also "super lice":** Karen Weintraub, "Revenge of the Super Lice," *Scientific American* 316, no. 6 (2017): 24–25.

50 **specialized nitpicking comb:** Kosta Y. Mumcuoglu et al., "International Recommendations for an Effective Control of Head Louse Infestations," *International Journal of Dermatology* 60, no. 3 (2021): 272–80, https://doi.org10.1111/ijd.15096.

50 **on well-conditioned hair:** Mumcuoglu et al., "International Recommendations."

50 **prescribe stronger medicines:** Wendy L. Sanchezruiz, Donald S. Nuzum, and Samir A. Kouzi, "Oral Ivermectin for the Treatment of Head Lice Infestation," *Bulletin of the American Society of Hospital Pharmacists* 75, no. 13 (2018): 937–43, https://doi.org10.2146/ajhp170464.

50 **starve the lice:** "Head Lice: Treatment FAQs," Centers for Disease Control and

Prevention, last updated September 17, 2020, https://www.cdc.gov/parasites/lice/head/gen_info/faqs_treat.html.

51 **nits in your nethers:** E. Charles Osterberg et al., "Correlation between Pubic Hair Grooming and STIs: Results from a Nationally Representative Probability Sample," *Sexually Transmitted Infections* 93, no. 3 (2017): 162–66, https://doi.org10.1136/sextrans-2016-052687.

Head Hair & Body Hair

54 **that porcupine quills:** Gislene L. Gonçalves et al., "Divergent Genetic Mechanism Leads to Spiny Hair in Rodents," *PLoS One* 13, no. 8 (2018): e0202219, https://doi.org/10.1371/journal.pone.0202219.

54 **people evolved to lose most hair:** Nina G. Jablonski, *Skin: A Natural History* (Berkeley: University of California Press, 2019).

54 **from injury, infection:** Zia Sherrell, "What to Know about the Integumentary System," MedicalNewsToday, June 29, 2022, https://www.medicalnewstoday.com/articles/integumentary-system#how-it-works.

54 **cancer-causing UV rays:** Megan H. Trager et al., "Biomarkers in Melanoma and Non-Melanoma Skin Cancer Prevention and Risk Stratification," *Experimental Dermatology* 31, no. 1 (2022): 4–12, https://doi.org/10.1111/exd.14114.

54 **Regulating our body temperature:** Joyce Y. Kim and Harry Dao, "Physiology, Integument," StatPearls, last updated May 1, 2023, https://www.statpearls.com/point-of-care/29105.

54 **hairs are even more responsive to touch:** Emma H. Jönsson et al., "The Relation between Human Hair Follicle Density and Touch Perception," *Scientific Reports* 7, no. 1 (2017): 1–10.

54 **five million follicles:** Dmitri Wall et al., "Advances in Hair Growth," *Faculty Reviews* 11 (2022): 1, https://doi.org/10.12703/r/11-1.

54 **up to four strands:** Patrick M. Zito and Blake S. Raggio, "Hair Transplantation," National Library of Medicine, February 14, 2023.

54 **places on your body that never grow hair:** Ashley Tate, "6 Weird Places Where Body Hair Grows," Everyday Health, last updated November 25, 2013, https://www.everydayhealth.com/beauty-pictures/weird-places-where-body-hair-grows.aspx.

54 **scarred skin cannot grow hair:** Melanie Rodrigues et al., "Wound Healing: A Cellular Perspective," *Physiological Reviews* 99, no. 1 (2019): 665–706, https://doi.org/10.1152/physrev.00067.2017.

55 **it's already dead:** Kathryn Watson, "Is Hair Made of Dead Skin Cells?," Healthline, September 11, 2020, https://www.healthline.com/health/is-hair-dead.

55 **through a growing phase:** "Types of Hair Loss," NYU Langone Health, accessed January 9, 2024, https://nyulangone.org/conditions/hair-loss/types.

55 **rests in the follicle:** Sian Ferguson, "How Do Hair Follicles Function?," Healthline, last updated September 25, 2023, https://www.healthline.com/health/hair-follicle.

55 **stays in the growing phase:** Penelope A. Hirt and Ralf Paus, "Healthy Hair (Anatomy, Biology, Morphogenesis, Cycling, and Function)," in Maria Miteva, ed., *Alopecia* (Elsevier, 2019), https://doi.org/10.1016/b978-0-323-54825-0.00001-6.

55 **half an inch:** Morgan B. Murphrey, Sanjay Agarwal, and Patrick M. Zito, "Anatomy, Hair," StatPearls, last updated August 14, 2023, https://pubmed.ncbi.nlm.nih.gov/30020684/.

55 **grows faster in warmer months:** Gabriela Daniels, Ashiana Fraser, and Gillian E. Westgate, "How Different Is Human Hair? A Critical Appraisal of the Reported Differences in Global Hair Fibre Characteristics and Properties Towards Defining a More Relevant Framework for Hair Type Classification," *International Journal of Cosmetic Science* 45, no. 1 (2023): 50–61, https://doi.org/10.1111/ics.12819.

55 **Stress can affect hair growth:** Soraya Azzawi, Lauren R. Penzi, and Maryanne M. Senna, "Immune Privilege Collapse and Alopecia Development: Is Stress a Factor," *Skin Appendage Disorders* 4, no. 4 (2018): 236–44, https://doi.org/10.1159/000485080.

55 **and hair damage:** T. Grant Phillips, W. Paul Slomiany, and Robert Allison, "Hair Loss: Common Causes and Treatment," *American Family Physician* 96, no. 6 (2017): 371–78.

55 **resting growth phase:** Ezra Hoover, Mandy Alhajj, and Jose L. Flores, "Physiology, Hair," StatPearls, last updated July 30, 2023, https://www.ncbi.nlm.nih.gov/books/NBK499948/.

55 **Head hair has:** Murphrey, Agarwal, and Zito, "Anatomy, Hair."

55 **Beard hair can:** Jyoti Gupta et al., "A Comparative Study on the Rate of Anagen Effluvium and Survival Rates of Scalp, Beard, and Chest Hair in Hair Restoration Procedure of Scalp," *Journal of Cutaneous and Aesthetic Surgery* 12, no. 2 (2019): 118–23, https://doi.org/10.4103/jcas.jcas_49_18.

55 **eyelashes and eyebrows:** David Buckley, "Hair Loss and Hair Growth," in *Textbook of Primary Care Dermatology* (Springer, 2021): 347–59.

55 **four times faster:** Anagha Bangalore Kumar, Huma Shamim, and Umashankar Nagaraju, "Premature Graying of Hair: Review with Updates," *International Journal of Trichology* 10, no. 5 (2018): 198–203, https://doi.org/10.4103/ijt.ijt_47_18.

55 **Vellus hair is:** "What Is the Structure of Hair and How Does It Grow?," InformedHealth.org, August 29, 2019, https://www.ncbi.nlm.nih.gov/books/NBK546248/.

55 **into terminal hair:** Monika Grymowicz et al., "Hormonal Effects on Hair Follicles," *International Journal of Molecular Sciences* 21, no. 15 (2020): 5342, https://doi.org/10.3390/ijms21155342.

56 **Terminal hair is the thicker:** "Terminal Hair," Biology Online Dictionary, June 28, 2021, https://www.biologyonline.com/dictionary/terminal-hair.

56 **vellus hair can turn into terminal hair:** "What Is the Structure of Hair and How Does It Grow?" InformedHealth.org.

56 **mustaches and beards:** Grymowicz et al., "Hormonal Effects on Hair Follicles."

56 **less than a third:** Heather L. Brannon, "Terminal Hair: Puberty Growth Phases from Vellus Hair," Verywell Health, last updated October 26, 2022, https://www.verywellhealth.com/terminal-hair-1069284.

57 **chin and upper lip:** Emilia Javorsky et al., "Race, Rather Than Skin Pigmentation, Predicts Facial Hair Growth in Women," *Journal of Clinical and Aesthetic Dermatology* 7, no. 5 (2014): 24.

57 **like polycystic ovary syndrome:** Ricardo Azziz, "Polycystic Ovary Syndrome," *Obstetrics and Gynecology* 132, no. 2 (2018): 321–36, https://doi.org/10.1097/AOG.0000000000002698.

57 **gender-affirming hormone therapy:** Guy T'Sjoen et al., "Endocrinology of

Transgender Medicine," *Endocrine Reviews* 40, no. 1 (2019): 97–117, https://doi.org/10.1210/er.2018-00011.

57 **body hair thickening:** Mia J. Bertoli et al., "Female Pattern Hair Loss: A Comprehensive Review," *Dermatologic Therapy* 33, no. 6 (2020): e14055, https://doi.org/10.1111/dth.14055.

57 **take feminizing hormones:** Kevin R. Brough and Rochelle R. Torgerson, "Hormonal Therapy in Female Pattern Hair Loss," *International Journal of Women's Dermatology* 3, no. 1 (2017): 53–57, https://doi.org/10.1016/j.ijwd.2017.01.001.

57 **change your scalp hair:** Grymowicz et al., "Hormonal Effects on Hair Follicles."

57 **born blond but turn:** Magdalena Kukla-Bartoszek et al., "Investigating the Impact of Age-Depended Hair Colour Darkening during Childhood on DNA-Based Hair Colour Prediction with the HIrisPlex System," *Forensic Science International: Genetics* 36 (2018): 26–33, https://doi.org/10.1016/j.fsigen.2018.06.007.

57 **supertight coils after puberty:** Gillian E. Westgate, Rebecca S. Ginger, and Martin R. Green, "The Biology and Genetics of Curly Hair," *Experimental Dermatology* 26, no. 6 (2017): 483–90, https://doi.org/10.1111/exd.13347.

57 **various stages of life:** Grymowicz et al., "Hormonal Effects on Hair Follicles."

57 **than before chemotherapy:** Anupam Das, Abhishek De, and Subrata Malakar, "Disorders of Hair Cycle," in *IADVL Textbook of Trichology* (Jaypee Digital, 2018): 184.

57 **100,000 strands of hair:** Murphrey, Agarwal, and Zito, "Anatomy, Hair."

58 **means "itch-dirt":** K. M. Uma Kumari, Narayan Prasad Yadav, and Suaib Luqman, "Promising Essential Oils/Plant Extracts in the Prevention and Treatment of Dandruff Pathogenesis," *Current Topics in Medicinal Chemistry* 22, no. 13 (2022): 1104–33, https://doi.org/10.2174/1568026622666220531120226.

58 **Dry dandruff is:** Jayata S. Mawani, Suraj N. Mali, and Amit P. Pratap, "Formulation and Evaluation of Antidandruff Shampoo Using Mannosylerythritol Lipid (MEL) as a Bio-Surfactant," *Tenside Surfactants Detergents* 60, no. 1 (2023): 44–53, https://doi.org/10.1515/tsd-2022-2449.

58 **dandruff becomes "wet":** Angelica Bottaro, "How to Get Rid of Wet Dandruff," Verywell Health, last updated October 25, 2023, https://www.verywellhealth.com/wet-dandruff-treatment-5197087.

58 **Dandruff can happen:** Yvette Brazier, "How to Treat Dandruff," MedicalNewsToday, last updated April 21, 2023, https://www.medicalnewstoday.com/articles/152844.

58 **UV rays from sunlight might help:** "Dandruff: Diagnosis and Treatment," Mayo Clinic, last updated August 25, 2023, https://www.mayoclinic.org/diseases-conditions/dandruff/diagnosis-treatment/drc-20353854.

58 **but sun exposure:** Yönter Meray, Duygu Gençalp, and Mümtaz Güran, "Putting It All Together to Understand the Role of *Malassezia spp.* in Dandruff Etiology," *Mycopathologia* 183 (2018): 893–903, https://doi.org/10.1007/s11046-018-0283-4.

58 **more common in the winter:** Mayada Kamel Mohammed, "Epidemiology of Dandruff and Effectiveness of Treatment among Tikrit Medical College Students," *Systematic Reviews in Pharmacy* 11, no. 3 (2020): 786–90, https://doi.org/10.31838/srp.2020.3.109.

58 **dried leftover hair products:** James Roland, "What Type of Dandruff Is Causing Your Flaky Scalp?" Healthline, last updated

January 8, 2021, https://www.healthline.com/health/types-of-dandruff.

58 **Scientists believe that a scalp fungus:** Sally G. Grimshaw et al., "The Diversity and Abundance of Fungi and Bacteria on the Healthy and Dandruff Affected Human Scalp," *PLoS One* 14, no. 12 (2019): e0225796, https://doi.org/10.1371/journal.pone.0225796.

58 **Coconut oil is a natural:** Rituja Saxena et al., "Longitudinal Study of the Scalp Microbiome Suggests Coconut Oil to Enrich Healthy Scalp Commensals," *Scientific Reports* 11, no. 1 (2021): 7220, https://doi.org/10.1038/s41598-021-86454-1.

59 **antifungal essential oils:** Ladislav Kokoska et al., "Plant-Derived Products as Antibacterial and Antifungal Agents in Human Health Care," *Current Medicinal Chemistry* 26, no. 29 (2019): 5501–41, https://doi.org/10.2174/0929867325666180831144344.

59 **suggest additional treatments:** "Scalp Psoriasis: Shampoos, Scale Softeners, and Other Treatments," American Academy of Dermatology Association, accessed January 9, 2024, https://www.aad.org/public/diseases/psoriasis/treatment/genitals/scalp-shampoo.

59 **seborrheic dermatitis, which:** Stephanie Watson, "Scalp Problems," WebMD, last updated September 18, 2023, https://www.webmd.com/skin-problems-and-treatments/scalp-problems.

59 **Dandruff, psoriasis, and seborrheic dermatitis:** Heba Hassan Ali Muhammad, Manal Mohamed Elsayed, and Mohamed Ibrahim Elghareeb, "Brief Overview about Topical Treatment of Psoriasis and Seborrheic Dermatitis," *Journal of Pharmaceutical Negative Results* 13, no. 7 (2022): 4785–91.

59 **half of all people:** Eulalia Peri et al., "No Itching or Flaking—Just a Naturally Healthy Scalp," *South African Pharmaceutical and Cosmetic Review* 47, no. 2 (2020): 34–40, https://hdl.handle.net/10520/ejc-im_sapcr-v47-n2-a9.

59 **a hundred and fifty hairs each day:** Moteb Kalaf Alotaibi, "Telogen Effluvium: A Review," *International Journal of Medicine in Developing Countries* 3 (2019): 797–801, https://doi.org/10.24911/IJMDC.51-1544654026.

59 **hair falls out more than usual:** Phillips, Slomiany, and Allison, "Hair Loss."

59 **Illness and certain medications:** Sumit Sethi, "Hair and Nail Disorders," in Rashmi Sarkar, ed., *Concise Dermatology* (CRC Press, 2021), 233–41.

60 **like alopecia areata:** Paul Ludmann, "Hair Loss Types: Alopecia Areata Overview," American Academy of Dermatology Association, last updated August 30, 2023, https://www.aad.org/public/diseases/hair-loss/types/alopecia.

60 **masculinizing gender-affirming hormones:** Julia L. Gao et al., "Androgenetic Alopecia in Transgender and Gender Diverse Populations: A Review of Therapeutics," *Journal of the American Academy of Dermatology* 89, no. 4 (2021): 774–83, https://doi.org/10.1016/j.jaad.2021.08.067.

60 **called androgenetic alopecia:** Lauren C. Strazzulla et al., "Alopecia Areata: Disease Characteristics, Clinical Evaluation, and New Perspectives on Pathogenesis," *Journal of the American Academy of Dermatology* 78, no. 1 (2018): 1–12, https://doi.org/10.1016/j.jaad.2017.04.1141.

60 **hair follicles shrink:** Nicholas John Sadgrove, "The 'Bald' Phenotype (Androgenetic Alopecia) Is Caused by the High Glycaemic, High Cholesterol and Low Mineral 'Western Diet,'" *Trends in*

Food Science and Technology 116 (2021): 1170–78, https://doi.org/10.1016/j.tifs.2021.06.056.

60 **even if it's an autoimmune disease:** Jane E. Brody, "She Was Losing Fistfuls of Hair. But What Was Causing It?," *New York Times*, February 3, 2020, https://www.nytimes.com/2020/02/03/well/live/she-was-losing-fistfuls-of-hair-what-was-causing-it.html.

60 **silk or satin pillowcase:** Lacey Muinos, "14 Best Pillowcases for Hair and Skin," Healthline, September 30, 2022, https://www.healthline.com/health/skin/pillowcases-for-hair-and-skin.

60 **wash it too much:** Ralph M. Trüeb et al., "Scalp Condition Impacts Hair Growth and Retention Via Oxidative Stress," *International Journal of Trichology* 10, no. 6 (2018): 262–70, https://doi.org/10.4103/ijt.ijt_57_18.

61 **dry or low-porosity hair:** Rachel Nall, "How to Care for Low Porosity Hair," Healthline, September 12, 2019, https://www.healthline.com/health/low-porosity-hair.

61 **Split ends usually:** Wen Yang et al., "On the Strength of Hair across Species," *Matter* 2, no. 1 (2020): 136–49, https://doi.org/10.1016/j.matt.2019.09.019.

61 **hair reacts differently:** Simone Marie, "6 Surprising Causes of Frizzy Hair—and 8 Ways to Combat It," Healthline, June 3, 2021, https://www.healthline.com/health/beauty-skin-care/what-causes-frizzy-hair.

61 **weather can cause hair:** Bee Shapiro, "Dry Winter Hair Is the Worst," *New York Times*, February 20, 2018. https://www.nytimes.com/2018/02/20/style/dry-winter-hair-solutions.html.

61 **One or more sharp blades:** Kevin Cowley et al., "Blade Shaving," in Zoe Diana Draelos, ed., *Cosmetic Dermatology: Products and Procedures* (Wiley, 2022), 223–30,

https://onlinelibrary.wiley.com/doi/book/10.1002/9781119676881.

61 **regrowth (called stubble):** Adebola Ogunbiyi, "Pseudofolliculitis Barbae; Current Treatment Options," *Clinical, Cosmetic and Investigational Dermatology* 12 (2019): 241–47, https://doi.org/10.2147/CCID.S149250.

62 **avoid razor burn:** Thanisorn Sukakul et al., "Facial Hair Shaving Behavior and Skin Problems of Shaved Areas of Males," *Journal of Dermatology* 48, no. 9 (2021): 1409–13, https://doi.org/10.1111/1346-8138.16034.

62 **Trimming eliminates the risk:** Eloise Galligan et al., "A Cut Above the Rest: Trimming as a Painless Depilatory," *Pediatric Dermatology* 36, no. 5 (2019): 753–54, https://doi.org/10.1111/pde.13938.

63 **other hair-removal methods:** Galligan et al., "A Cut Above the Rest."

63 **Hair-removal potions are chemical compounds:** Kenneth Morris, "Depilatories, Masks, Scrubs and Bleaching Preparations," in *Poucher's Perfumes, Cosmetics and Soaps*, vol. 3, *Cosmetics* (Springer, 1993): 91–108.

63 **skin feels smoother:** Zoe Kececioglu Draelos, "Cosmetics: An Overview," *Current Problems in Dermatology* 7, no. 2 (1995): 45–64, https://doi.org/10.1016/S1040-0486(09)80017-3.

63 **cause rashes and burns:** Eirlys Roberts, "Chemistry and the Consumer," *Royal Institute of Chemistry, Reviews* 1, no. 1 (1968): 1–12.

63 **plucking or tweezing:** Corey Whelan, "All about Plucking Hair: The Good, the Bad, and the Painful," Healthline, July 23, 2020, https://www.healthline.com/health/all-about-plucking-hair.

63 **root and all:** Heather L. Brannon, "Pros and Cons of 10 Hair Removal Methods,"

Verywell Health, last updated May 2, 2023, https://www.verywellhealth.com/hair-removal-methods-1068792.

63 **are called epilators:** Valencia Higuera, "Is an Epilator the Hair Remover You've Been Looking For?," Healthline, last updated April 14, 2023, https://www.healthline.com/health/epilator.

63 **improper tweezing can:** "How Tweezing Unwanted Hair Can Damage Your Skin," Hair.com by L'Oréal, accessed January 4, 2024, https://www.hair.com/can-plucking-and-tweezing-hair-damage-skin.html.

63 **speedier version of tweezing:** Victoria Sherrow, *Encyclopedia of Hair: A Cultural History* (ABC-CLIO, 2023).

64 **smoother for longer:** Naomi Torres, "Hair Threading 101," *Byrdie*, February 21, 2022, https://www.byrdie.com/threading-hair-removal-101-1717114#toc-benefits-of-threading.

64 **any other complications:** Subodh Verma, "Eyebrow Threading: A Popular Hair-Removal Procedure and Its Seldom-Discussed Complications," *Clinical and Experimental Dermatology* 34, no. 3 (2009): 363–65, https://doi.org/10.1111/j.1365-2230.2008.02920.x.

64 **Beeswax is one:** A. L. Rowser, *Ethical Beauty Products* (New York: Rosen Publishing, 2020).

64 **"Soft" wax requires:** Won-Jin Baek and Chae-Jeong Han, "The Effect of Pursuit Benefit of Beauty Waxing on Reuse Intention," *Journal of Convergence for Information Technology* 10, no. 9 (2020): 244–50.

64 **top layer of dead skin cells:** Mohammed Al-Haddab et al., "The Effect of Waxing Versus Shaving on the Efficacy of Laser Hair Removal," *Dermatologic Surgery* 43, no. 4 (2017): 548–52, https://doi.org/10.1097/DSS.0000000000001025.

64 **bleaching doesn't remove hair:** Katie McCarthy, "How to Bleach Facial and Body Hair, According to Skin Experts," *Byrdie*, November 24, 2021, https://www.byrdie.com/bleaching-facial-and-body-hair-101-1716732.

64 **allergic to bleaching:** K. Forster et al., "Hair Bleaching and Skin Burning," *Annals of Burns and Fire Disasters* 25, no. 4 (2012): 200–202, https://www.ncbi.nlm.nih.gov/pmc/articles/PMC3664529/.

65 **techniques like electrolysis, light therapy, and laser treatments:** Tanvi Vaidya, Marc H. Hohman, and D. Dinesh Kumar, "Laser Hair Removal," StatPearls, last updated March 1, 2023, https://www.ncbi.nlm.nih.gov/books/NBK507861/.

65 **licensed professionals like dermatologists and estheticians:** Rebecca Strong, "What's the Difference between an Esthetician and a Dermatologist?," Healthline, May 2, 2022, https://www.healthline.com/health/beauty-skincare/esthetician-vs-dermatologist.

65 **removal is permanent:** Kristeen Cherney, "Laser Hair Removal: Permanent or Temporary Fix?" Healthline, last updated June 16, 2018, https://www.healthline.com/health/beauty-skin-care/is-laser-hair-removal-permanent.

65 **prone to scarring:** "African American Skin Treatment and Dermatology NYC," Dr. Michele Green, MD, accessed January 9, 2024, https://www.michelegreenmd.com/african-american-skin-treatment-dermatology.

65 **retreat back into their follicles:** Albert Einstein, "Dermatologic Pathologies," in Susan G. Salvo, *Mosby's Pathology for Massage Therapists*, 4th ed., VitalSource eBook (Elsevier, 2017), 73.

65 **known as razor bumps:** Brooke Schleehauf, "6 Razor Bump Prevention Tips from

Dermatologists," American Academy of Dermatology Association, last updated October 3, 2022, https://www.aad.org /public/everyday-care/skin-care-basics /hair/razor-bump-prevention.

66 **Ingrown hairs or folliculitis:** Richard D. Winters and Mark Mitchell, "Folliculitis," StatPearls, last updated August 8, 2023, https://www.statpearls.com/point-of -care/21873.

66 **poorly handled ingrown hairs and folliculitis:** Murat Durdu et al., "High Accuracy of Recognition of Common Forms of Folliculitis by Dermoscopy: An Observational Study," *Journal of the American Academy of Dermatology* 81, no. 2 (2019): 463–71, https://doi .org/10.1016/j.jaad.2019.03.054.

66 **Gentle exfoliation helps:** Radhika Parasuram Rajam, Sivaranjani Kannan, and Deepa Kajendran, "Cosmeceuticals: An Emerging Technology—A Review," *World Journal of Pharmaceutical Research* 8, no. 12 (2019): 664–85, https://doi .org/10.20959/wjpr201912-16162.

66 **wigs called merkins:** Jonathan Faiers, *Fur: A Sensitive History* (Yale University Press, 2020).

66 **is called trichotillomania:** Katharine Anne Phillips and Dan J. Stein, "Trichotillomania," Merck Manuals Professional Version, last updated June 2023, https://www.merck manuals.com/professional/psychiatric -disorders/obsessive-compulsive-and -related-disorders/trichotillomania.

66 **ten and thirteen years of age:** Emily D. Henkel, Sasha D. Jaquez, and Lucia Z. Diaz, "Pediatric Trichotillomania: Review of Management," *Pediatric Dermatology* 36, no. 6 (2019): 803–807, https://doi .org/10.1111/pde.13954.

66 **up to 1 out of every 50:** Gregory J. Everett, Mohammad Jafferany, and Jonathon

Skurya, "Recent Advances in the Treatment of Trichotillomania (Hair-Pulling Disorder)," *Dermatologic Therapy* 33, no. 6 (2020): e13818, https://doi.org/10.1111/dth.13818.

66 **also have dermatillomania:** Jon E. Grant and Samuel R. Chamberlain, "Characteristics of 262 Adults with Skin Picking Disorder," *Comprehensive Psychiatry* 117 (2022): 152338, https://doi .org/10.1016/j.comppsych.2022.152338.

67 **the obsessive-compulsive spectrum:** Aubree D. Pereyra, and Abdolreza Saadabadi, "Trichotillomania," StatPearls, last updated June 26, 2023, https://www .ncbi.nlm.nih.gov/books/NBK493186 /#_article-30593_s11.

Chests & Breasts

70 **grow milk-producing breasts:** "TPWD: Mammal Scrabble," Texas Parks and Wildlife, accessed January 9, 2024, https://tpwd.texas.gov/publications /nonpwdpubs/young_naturalist/animals /mammal_scrabble.

70 **develop permanent breasts:** Nathaniel Lee, David Anderson, and Jessica Orwig, "The Science of Why Human Breasts Are So Big," *Business Insider*, November 9, 2018, https://www.businessinsider.com/why -are-human-breasts-big-2018-2.

70 **born with flat chests:** Yusuf S. Khan and Hussain Sajjad, "Anatomy, Thorax, Mammary Gland," StatPearls, last updated July 24, 2023, https://www.ncbi.nlm.nih .gov/books/NBK547666.

70 **tiny tube-like milk ducts:** "General Breast Health," Stony Brook University Hospital, accessed January 9, 2024, https://www .stonybrookmedicine.edu/patientcare /breasthealth.

70 **Estrogen also matures:** "Normal Breast Development," Stanford Medicine Children's Health, accessed January 9,

2024, https://www.stanfordchildrens.org/en/topic/default?id=normal-breast-development-90-P01624.

70 **increases muscle mass:** Ann Pietrangelo, "How Testosterone Benefits Your Body," Healthline, last updated September 18, 2018, https://www.healthline.com/health/benefits-testosterone.

71 **size of their chest:** Hannah L. Quittkat et al., "Body Dissatisfaction, Importance of Appearance, and Body Appreciation in Men and Women over the Lifespan," *Frontiers in Psychiatry* 10 (2019): 864, https://doi.org/10.3389/fpsyt.2019.00864.

71 **muscles they're concerned about:** Viren Swami et al., "The Breast Size Satisfaction Survey (BSSS): Breast Size Dissatisfaction and Its Antecedents and Outcomes in Women from 40 Nations," *Body Image* 32 (2020): 199–217, https://doi.org/10.1016/j.bodyim.2020.01.006.

72 **or unexpected breasts:** Ronald S. Swerdloff and Jason C. M. Ng, "Gynecomastia: Etiology, Diagnosis, and Treatment," Endotext, last updated January 6, 2023, https://www.ncbi.nlm.nih.gov/books/NBK279105/.

72 **with congenital athelia:** "Congenital Athelia," Children's Health, accessed January 9, 2024, https://www.childrens.com/specialties-services/conditions/athelia.

72 **known as polythelia:** Nirupama De Silva, "Pediatric Polythelia," Children's Health, accessed January 9, 2024, https://www.childrens.com/specialties-services/conditions/polythelia.

72 **is called polymastia:** Seong Bae Hwang et al., "Accessory Axillary Breast Excision with Liposuction Using Minimal Incision: A Preliminary Report," *Aesthetic Plastic Surgery* 41, no. 1 (2017): https://doi.org/10–18, 10.1007/s00266-016-0729-3.

72 **extra nipples are also associated:** Steffi Mayer et al., "Breast Disorders in Children and Adolescents," in Prem Puri and Michael E. Höllwarth, eds., *Pediatric Surgery: Diagnosis and Management* (Springer International Publishing, 2023), 405–12.

72 **Every size and shape:** Jasmine Shaikh, "How Big Are Areolas Usually?," MedicineNet, last updated December 11, 2020, https://www.medicinenet.com/how_big_are_areolas_usually/article.htm.

73 **called Montgomery's glands:** Ashley Alex, Eva Bhandary, and Kandace P. McGuire, "Anatomy and Physiology of the Breast during Pregnancy and Lactation," in Sadaf Alipour and Ramesh Omranipour, eds., *Diseases of the Breast during Pregnancy and Lactation* (Springer, 2020), 3–7.

73 **amount of antibacterial oil:** Alex, Bhandary, and McGuire, "Anatomy and Physiology."

73 **Nipples also come in all:** Laura Barcella, "What's Your Nipple Type? And 24 Other Nipple Facts," Healthline, last updated February 7, 2023, https://www.healthline.com/health/nipple-facts-male-and-female.

74 **Most people's nipples protrude:** Serenity Mirabito, "Different Types of Nipples: What You Need to Know," Verywell Health, last updated March 21, 2023, https://www.verywellhealth.com/nipple-variations-430664.

74 **When a nipple chafes:** Renato Marchiori Bakos et al., "Dermatology and Sports," in *Dermatology in Public Health Environments: A Comprehensive Textbook* (Springer, 2023), 1429–38.

74 **from "runner's nipple":** Brooke R. Brisbine et al., "The Occurrence, Causes and Perceived Performance Effects of Breast Injuries in Elite Female Athletes," *Journal of Sports Science and Medicine* 18, no. 3

(2019): 569, https://www.ncbi.nlm.nih.gov /pmc/articles/PMC6683617/.

74 **neutralize nipple chafing:** Stephanie Watson, "Understanding Nipple Pain: Causes, Treatment, and More," Healthline, last updated April 24, 2023, https:// www.healthline.com/health/why-do-my -nipples-hurt.

75 **Up to 1 in every 5:** Deepti Nagaraja Rao and Ryan Winters, "Inverted Nipple," StatPearls, last updated July 4, 2023. https://www .ncbi.nlm.nih.gov/books/NBK563190.

75 **may experience galactorrhea:** Richard D. Bruehlman, Stella Winters, and Connor McKittrick, "Galactorrhea: Rapid Evidence Review," *American Family Physician* 106, no. 6 (2022): 695–700.

75 **can cause nipple discharge:** "Nipple Discharge." Mayo Clinic, December 4, 2021, https://www.mayoclinic.org/symptoms /nipple-discharge/basics/causes/sym -20050946.

75 **sign of breast cancer:** Su-Ju Lee et al., "ACR Appropriateness Criteria Evaluation of Nipple Discharge," *Journal of the American College of Radiology* 14, no. 5, suppl. (2017): S138–S153, https://doi .org/10.1016/j.jacr.2017.01.030.

76 **feel sore or itchy:** "Why Are My Breasts Sore?," Nemours Teen Health, July 2019, https://kidshealth.org/en/teens/sore -breasts.html.

76 **alternating hot and cold compresses:** "Why Are My Breasts Sore?"

76 **If chest pain doesn't go away:** Muhammad T. Tahir and Shafeek Shamsudeen, "Mastalgia," StatPearls, last updated November 1, 2022, https://www .ncbi.nlm.nih.gov/books/NBK562195.

76 **become more muscular:** Taline Santos Da Costa et al., "Influence of Biological Maturity on the Muscular Strength

of Young Male and Female Swimmers," *Journal of Human Kinetics* 78 (2021): 67–77, https://doi.org/10.2478/hukin -2021-0029.

76 **your pectoralis muscles:** Khan and Sajjad, "Anatomy, Thorax, Mammary Gland."

77 **pecs that easily puff up:** Stephen M. Roth, "Genetic Aspects of Skeletal Muscle Strength and Mass with Relevance to Sarcopenia," *Bonekey Reports* 1 (2012): 58, https://doi.org/10.1038/bonekey.2012.58.

77 **can encourage unrealistic:** Veya Seekis, Graham Leslie Bradley, and Amanda Louise Duffy, "Social Networking Sites and Men's Drive for Muscularity: Testing a Revised Objectification Model," *Psychology of Men and Masculinity* 2, no. 1: 189–200, https:// doi.org/10.1037/men0000265.

77 **also known as bigorexia:** Karen M. Skemp, Renae L. Elwood, and David M. Reineke, "Adolescent Boys Are at Risk for Body Image Dissatisfaction and Muscle Dysmorphia," *Californian Journal of Health Promotion* 17, no. 1 (2019): 61–70, https:// doi.org/10.32398/cjhp.v17i1.2224.

77 **disconnect between the person's:** Silvia Cerea et al., "Muscle Dysmorphia and Its Associated Psychological Features in Three Groups of Recreational Athletes," *Scientific Reports* 8, no. 1 (2018): 8877, https://doi .org/10.1038/s41598-018-27176-9.

77 **suffering from bigorexia:** Almut Zeeck et al., "Muscle Dysmorphic Disorder Inventory (MDDI): Validation of a German Version with a Focus on Gender," *PLoS ONE* 13 (11): e0207535, https://doi.org/10.1371/journal .pone.0207535.

78 **thoughts take over your life:** US Substance Abuse and Mental Health Services Administration, "Table 23, DSM-IV to DSM-5 Body Dysmorphic Disorder Comparison—DSM-5 Changes," https://

www.ncbi.nlm.nih.gov/books/NBK519712
/table/ch3.t19/.

78 **look healthy on the outside:** David Tod, Christian Edwards, and Ieuan Cranswick, "Muscle Dysmorphia: Current Insights," *Psychology Research and Behavior Management* 9 (August): 179–88, https://doi.org/10.2147/prbm.s97404.

78 **time to stretch properly:** "Stretch Marks," Cleveland Clinic, last updated May 4, 2022, https://my.clevelandclinic.org/health /articles/10785-stretch-marks.

78 **referred to as striae gravidarum:** B. Farahnik et al., "Striae Gravidarum: Risk Factors, Prevention, and Management," *International Journal of Women's Dermatology* 3, no. 2 (2017): 77–85.

78 **very common chest condition:** Girish Sharma and Yvonne M. Carter, "Pectus Excavatum," StatPearls, last updated July 17, 2023, https://www.ncbi.nlm.nih .gov/books/NBK430918/.

78 **five times more likely:** Irene T. Ma et al., "Pectus Excavatum in Adult Women," *Plastic and Reconstructive Surgery* 135, no. 2 (2015): 303e–312e, https://doi .org/10.1097/prs.0000000000000990

79 **visible breast tissue:** "Gynecomastia: Etiology, Diagnosis, and Treatment," Endotext, January 6, 2023, https://www .ncbi.nlm.nih.gov/books/NBK279105/.

79 **intersex variations assigned male:** Darius Haghighat et al., "Intersex People's Perspectives on Affirming Healthcare Practices: A Qualitative Study," *Social Science and Medicine* 329 (2023): 116047, https://doi.org/10.1016 /j.socscimed.2023.116047.

80 **areola and nipple point downward:** Amaury A. Martinez and Susan Chung, "Breast Ptosis," StatPearls, last updated November 12, 2023, https://www.ncbi.nlm .nih.gov/books/NBK567792/.

80 **Pendulous breasts are:** "What to Know about Sagging Breasts," WebMD, May 27, 2021. https://www.webmd.com/women /what-to-know-about-sagging-breasts.

80 **body's overall tone:** Nicole Davis, "Try This: 13 Breast-Firming Exercises," Healthline, last updated April 17, 2023, https://www .healthline.com/health/fitness-exercise /breast-firming-exercises.

80 **illusion of breast perkiness:** "What to Know about Sagging Breasts," WebMD.

81 **areola and nipple darkening:** "Normal Breast Development and Changes," Johns Hopkins Medicine, July 20, 2020, https:// www.hopkinsmedicine.org/health /conditions-and-diseases/normal-breast -development-and-changes.

81 **breast growth can happen:** Jennifer L. Bercaw-Pratt and Jennifer E. Dietrich, "Breast Development," Texas Children's Hospital, https://www.texaschildrens.org /health/breast-development.

81 **very athletic people:** Diana Zuckerman and Sarah Romano, "Girls and Sports," National Center for Health Research, January 28, 2021, http://www.center4research.org /female-athletes/.

81 **development may restart:** Shane A. Norris et al., "Nutrition in Adolescent Growth and Development," *The Lancet* 399, no. 10320 (2022): 172–84, https://doi.org/10.1016 /S0140-6736(21)01590-7.

81 **not make a significant difference:** Corey Whelan, "Can You Increase Your Breast Size by Eating Certain Foods?," Healthline, July 16, 2020, https://www.healthline.com /health/can-you-increase-your-breast -size-by-eating-certain-foods#what -determines-breast-size.

82 **larger than the other:** Kiara Anthony, "Breast Asymmetry," Healthline, last updated September 29, 2018, https://

www.healthline.com/health/breast
-asymmetry#causes.

82 **smaller breast "catches up":** Tracee
Cornforth, "Why Are My Breasts Uneven?,"
Verywell Health, last updated October 13,
2023, https://www.verywellhealth.com
/one-breast-bigger-than-other-3969225.

82 **Uneven breasts are sometimes a sign:**
Norma I. Cruz and Leo Corchin, "Breast
Asymmetry Pattern in Women with
Idiopathic Scoliosis," *Boletín de la
Asociación Médica de Puerto Rico* 105,
no. 3: 9–12.

83 **Big breasts can cause pain:** Myint Oo et al.,
"Relationship between Brassiere Cup Size
and Shoulder-Neck Pain in Women," *Open
Orthopaedics Journal* 6, no. 1: 140–42,
https://doi.org/10.2174/187432500120601
0140.

83 **help support heavy breasts:** Whelan, "Can
You Increase Your Breast Size?"

83 **itchy, painful, and even smelly rash:** Susan
York Morris, "Why Is There a Rash under
My Breast?," Healthline, last updated
February 23, 2023, https://www.healthline
.com/health/skin-disorders/rash-under
-breast#causes.

83 **perfect breeding ground:** Morris, "Why Is
There a Rash?"

83 **poorly fitting bra:** Jody Amable, "5 Signs
Your Bra Is Definitely Too Tight—and How
to Find Your Perfect Size," Healthline,
October 30, 2020, https://www.healthline
.com/health/tight-bra.

83 **help heal irritated skin:** Jessica Toscano,
"How to Survive Boob Sweat Season," *Self*,
June 7, 2022, https://www.self.com/story
/boob-sweat.

83 **A breast reduction is considered:** Richard
Greco and Barrett Noone, "Evidence-
Based Medicine: Reduction Mammaplasty,"
Plastic and Reconstructive Surgery 139,

no. 1 (2017): 230e–239e, https://doi.org/
10.1097/PRS.0000000000002856.

84 **can get "top surgery":** "Masculinizing
Surgery," Mayo Clinic, January 13, 2022,
https://www.mayoclinic.org/tests
-procedures/top-surgery-for-transgender
-men/about/pac-20469462.

85 **few lumps in your breast:** "Breast Lumps:
Causes and When to Call a Doctor,"
WebMD, last updated March 24, 2023,
https://www.webmd.com/breast-cancer
/guide/benign-breast-lumps.

85 **could feel abnormally lumpy:** "Breast
Lumps," WebMD.

85 **common noncancerous issues:** "Breast
Lumps," City of Hope, August 28, 2023,
https://www.cancercenter.com/cancer
-types/breast-cancer/diagnosis-and
-detection/breast-lumps.

85 **show up around puberty:** "Fibroadenoma,"
Mayo Clinic, October 13, 2022, https://
www.mayoclinic.org/diseases-conditions
/fibroadenoma/symptoms-causes/syc
-20352752.

86 **Harmless, fluid-filled sacs:** "Breast Cysts,"
Mayo Clinic, January 17, 2023, https://
www.mayoclinic.org/diseases-conditions
/breast-cysts/symptoms-causes/syc
-20370284.

86 **lumps felt during menstruation:**
"Premenstrual Breast Changes," Mount
Sinai Health System, last updated April 19,
2022, https://www.mountsinai.org/health
-library/symptoms/premenstrual-breast
-changes.

86 **being "breast aware":** "Breast Self-
Awareness," Johns Hopkins Medicine,
August 2, 2021, https://www.hopkins
medicine.org/health/wellness-and
-prevention/breast-self-awareness.

86 **lower the risk of:** Ashley Drohan et
al., "Breast Cancer after Reduction

Mammoplasty: A Population-Based Analysis of Incidence, Treatment, and Screening Patterns," *Journal of Clinical Oncology* 40, 16_suppl: e18785, https://doi.org/10.1200/jco.2022.40.16_suppl.e18785.

86 **cancer, it's still possible:** Jill P. Stone, Rebecca L. Hartley, and Claire Temple-Oberle, "Breast Cancer in Transgender Patients: A Systematic Review. Part 2: Female to Male," *European Journal of Surgical Oncology* 44, no. 10: 1463–68, https://doi.org/10.1016/j.ejso.2018.06.021.

87 **a history of breast cancer:** Sharon H. Giordano, "Breast Cancer in Men," *New England Journal of Medicine* 378, no. 24 (2018): 2311–20, https://doi.org/10.1056/NEJMra1707939.

87 **gender-affirming hormone therapy:** Christel J. M. De Blok et al., "Breast Cancer Risk in Transgender People Receiving Hormone Treatment: Nationwide Cohort Study in the Netherlands," *BMJ* 365 (2019): l1652, doi: 10.1136/bmj.l1652.

87 **Study your breasts carefully:** "Self-Examination Procedures," Stony Brook Cancer Center, accessed January 9, 2024, https://cancer.stonybrookmedicine.edu/breast-cancer-team/patients/bse/self-exam-procedures.

87 **three direction techniques:** "Self-Examination Procedures."

88 **same time every month:** "Breast Self-Exam," National Breast Cancer Foundation, June 2023, https://www.nationalbreastcancer.org/breast-self-exam/.

88 **if you ever have an issue:** "Breast Self-Exam," Cleveland Clinic, last updated June 7, 2023, https://my.clevelandclinic.org/health/diagnostics/3990-breast-self-exam.

88 **under the age of thirty:** Jacquelyn Cafasso, "Everything You Should Know about Breast Cancer in Your 20s and 30s," Healthline, last updated April 20, 2023, https://www.healthline.com/health/breast-cancer/breast-cancer-20s-30s.

88 **rare but not impossible:** Santhi D. Konduri et al., "Epidemiology of Male Breast Cancer," *Breast* 54 (2020): 8–14, https://doi.org/10.1016/j.breast.2020.08.010.

89 **person with limited mobility:** Cheryl Crow, "Adaptive Clothing for Disabilities and Body Differences," EverydayHealth.com, September 14, 2022, https://www.everydayhealth.com/healthy-living/adaptive-clothing-for-disabilities-and-body-differences/.

89 **behave like a good friend:** Talia Abbas, "11 Expert Tips for Finding the Right Bra Size and Fit." *Self*, July 23, 2018, https://www.self.com/story/tips-for-finding-the-right-bra-size-and-fit.

89 **Training bras, unlined:** Jennifer O'Donnell, "The Purpose of a Training Bra," Verywell Family, March 20, 2022, https://www.verywellfamily.com/what-is-a-training-bra-4017008.

90 **Padded bras have:** Allena Rissa, "Main Differences in Padded vs Non-Padded Bras," TheBetterFit, accessed January 9, 2024, https://thebetterfit.com/padded-vs-non-padded-bra/.

90 **Underwire bras have:** Chris Malbon et al., "The Effect of Underwired and Sports Bras on Breast Shape, Key Anthropometric Dimensions, and Body Armour Comfort," *Police Journal* 95, no. 3 (2022): 436–58, https://doi.org/10.1177/0032258X211011619.

90 **T-shirt bras are:** Allena Rissa, "What Is a T-Shirt Bra?" TheBetterFit, accessed January 9, 2024, https://thebetterfit.com/what-is-t-shirt-bra/.

90 **Push-up bras usually:** "Push-Up Bra History." LEAFtv, December 13, 2021, https://www.leaf.tv/articles/push-up-bra-history/.

90 **Bralettes usually have:** Allenna Rissa, "Wearing Bralettes Instead of Bras: How to Make the Transition," TheBetterFit, accessed January 9, 2024, https://thebetterfit.com/wearing-bralettes-instead-of-bras/#more-730.

90 **Bandeau bras usually:** Jené Luciani, *The Bra Book: An Intimate Guide to Finding the Right Bra, Shapewear, Swimsuit, and More!*, 2nd ed. (BenBella Books, 2017).

90 **Strapless bras are:** Luciani, *The Bra Book*.

90 **Bra tape is:** Amanda Oliver and Alexandria Taylor, "The Complete Beginner's Guide to Boob Tape," Reviewed, last updated October 2, 2023, https://reviewed.usatoday.com/style/features/boob-tape-guide.

90 **Minimizer bras usually:** Allena Rissa, "What Is a Minimizer Bra (And Should I Wear One)?" TheBetterFit, accessed January 9, 2024, accessed January 9, 2024, https://thebetterfit.com/what-is-minimizer-bra/.

91 **Sports bras are:** Allena Rissa, "Sports Bra vs Normal Bra [Key Differences]," TheBetterFit, accessed January 9, 2024, https://thebetterfit.com/sports-bra-vs-normal-bra/.

91 **going completely without:** Colleen Murphy, "What Effect Does Being Braless Have on My Body? Here's What Experts Say," *Health*, October 28, 2022.

91 **chest binders, kinesiology tape:** Sarah Peitzmeier et al., "Health Impact of Chest Binding among Transgender Adults: A Community-Engaged, Cross-Sectional Study," *Culture, Health and Sexuality* 19, no. 1: 64–75, https://doi.org/10.1080/13691058.2016.1191675.

91 **can be very confining:** Melissa Rorech and Adrien Ramirez, "What Is a Chest Binder and How Does It Work?," Reviewed, last updated May 25, 2022, https://reviewed.usatoday.com/health/features/what-is-chest-binder-how-does-it-work.

Bladders & Bowels

94 **medical terms for peeing and pooping:** Scott Mawer and Ali F. Alhawaj, "Physiology, Defecation," StatPearls, last updated November 13, 2023, https://www.ncbi.nlm.nih.gov/books/NBK539732/.

94 **extract all the nutrients:** Laura L. Azzouz and Sandeep Sharma, "Physiology, Large Intestine," StatPearls, last updated July 31, 2023, https://www.ncbi.nlm.nih.gov/books/NBK507857/.

94 **three times a day to three times a week:** Shuji Mitsuhashi et al., "Characterizing Normal Bowel Frequency and Consistency in a Representative Sample of Adults in the United States (NHANES)," *Official Journal of the American College of Gastroenterology* 113, no. 1 (2018): 115–23, https://doi.org/10.1038/ajg.2017.213.

94 **you may be constipated:** "Definition and Facts for Constipation," National Institute of Diabetes and Digestive and Kidney Diseases, last updated May 2018, https://www.niddk.nih.gov/health-information/digestive-diseases/constipation/definition-facts.

94 **chemical called stercobilin:** James X. Wu, Christian de Virgilio, and Danielle M. Hari, "New Onset of Painless Jaundice," in *Surgery: A Case Based Clinical Review*, 2nd ed. (Springer, 2020), 239–46.

95 **brown color. However,:** Pathipat Durongpongkasem, "Stool Color, Shape and Self Diagnosis," Samitivej, February 27, 2019, https://www.samitivejhospitals.com/article/detail/stool-color-blood-in-stool.

95 **liver trouble or a blockage:** Wu, de Virgilio, and Hari, "New Onset of Painless Jaundice."

95 **can cause green poop:** Minhthao Nguyen and Prasanna Tadi, "Iron Supplementation," StatPearls, last updated July 3, 2023, https://www.ncbi.nlm.nih.gov/books/NBK557376/.

96 **Diarrhea ranges from:** "Symptoms and Causes of Diarrhea," National Institute of Diabetes and Digestive and Kidney Diseases, last updated November 2016, https://www.niddk.nih.gov/health-information/digestive-diseases/diarrhea/symptoms-causes.

97 **causes of constipation:** Mojgan Foroutan, Nazila Bagheri, and Mohammad Darvishi, "Chronic Constipation: A Review of Literature," *Medicine* (Baltimore) 97, no. 20 (2018): e10631, https://doi.org/10.1097/MD.0000000000010631.

97 **half the population:** Robert S. Sandler and Anne F. Peery, "Rethinking What We Know about Hemorrhoids," *Clinical Gastroenterology and Hepatology* 17, no. 1 (2019): 8–15, https://doi.org/10.1016/j.cgh.2018.03.020.

97 **swollen veins in the rectum:** "Hemorrhoids," Mayo Clinic, August 25, 2023, https://www.mayoclinic.org/diseases-conditions/hemorrhoids/symptoms-causes/syc-20360268.

97 **can't see internal hemorrhoids:** "Hemorrhoids and What to Do about Them," Harvard Health, November 16, 2021, https://www.health.harvard.edu/diseases-and-conditions/hemorrhoids_and_what_to_do_about_them.

97 **One in ten people:** Sabrina Maria Ebinger et al., "Operative and Medical Treatment of Chronic Anal Fissures—A Review and Network Meta-Analysis of Randomized Controlled Trials," *Journal of Gastroenterology* 52 (2017): 663–76, https://doi.org/10.1007/s00535-017-1335-0.

98 **avoid bubble baths:** Ana Gotter, "How to Use Epsom Salt for Hemorrhoids," Healthline, February 1, 2019, https://www.healthline.com/health/epsom-salt-for-hemorrhoids#epsom-salt-bath.

98 **but rather anal warts:** "Anal Warts (Condyloma)," Cleveland Clinic, last updated September 2, 2022, https://my.clevelandclinic.org/health/diseases/24097-anal-warts.

98 **left untreated, they can spread:** "Genital HPV Infection—Basic Facts," Centers for Disease Control and Prevention, last updated April 12, 2022, https://www.cdc.gov/std/hpv/stdfact-hpv.htm.

98 **Stool testing can tell:** Karen J. Steffer et al., "The Practical Value of Comprehensive Stool Analysis in Detecting the Cause of Idiopathic Chronic Diarrhea," *Gastroenterology Clinics of North America* 41, no. 3 (2012): 539–60, https://doi.org/10.1016/j.gtc.2012.06.001.

98 **snoop your own poop:** Ziyuan Yang, Lu Leng, and Byung-Gyu Kim, "StoolNet for Color Classification of Stool Medical Images," *Electronics* 8, no. 12 (2019): 1464, https://doi.org/10.3390/electronics8121464.

99 **limit the spread of bacteria:** Nishant Aggarwal and Saran Lotfollahzadeh, "Recurrent Urinary Tract Infections," StatPearls, last updated on December 3, 2022, https://pubmed.ncbi.nlm.nih.gov/32491411/.

99 **twelve million Americans infected:** Peter J. Hotez and Cory Booker, "STOP: Study, Treat, Observe, and Prevent Neglected Diseases of Poverty Act," *PLoS Neglected Tropical Diseases* 14, no. 2 (2020): e0008064, https://doi.org/10.1371/journal.pntd.0008064.

99 **five and a half feet long:** Vanessa Romo, "Man Pulls 5½-Foot-Long Tapeworm out of His Body, Blames Sushi Habit," NPR, January 19, 2018, https://www.npr.org/sections/thetwo-way/2018/01/19/579130873/man-pulls-5-1-2-foot-long-tapeworm-out-of-his-body-blames-sushi-habit.

99 **lay eggs around the anus:** Ibraheem Ashankyty and Omar Hassan Amer, *Practical Manual for Detection of Parasites in Feces, Blood and Urine Samples* (Xlibris Corporation, 2020).

100 **spread from "toilet plumes":** Kathleen A. N. Aithinne et al., "Toilet Plume Aerosol Generation Rate and Environmental Contamination Following Bowl Water Inoculation with *Clostridium difficile* Spores," *American Journal of Infection Control* 47, no. 5 (2019): 515–20, https://doi.org/10.1016/j.ajic.2018.11.009.

100 **incorporating some of these tips:** Rachel Nall, "What Makes for a Typical Bowel Movement?," Healthline, last updated March 21, 2023, https://www.healthline.com/health/bowel-movement.

100 **longer the poop sits:** Jessica Caporuscio, "Why People Should Not Hold in Their Poop," MedicalNewsToday, last updated April 25, 2023, https://www.medicalnewstoday.com/articles/is-it-bad-to-hold-your-poop.

101 **Use a toilet stool:** Brian Krans, "Science Says Using a Squatty Potty Really Can Improve the Way You Poop," Healthline, February 3, 2019, https://www.healthline.com/health-news/science-says-toilet-footstools-really-can-improve-the-way-you-poop.

101 **Physical movement helps:** Debra Fulghum Bruce, "Exercise to Ease Constipation," WebMD, last updated August 11, 2022, https://www.webmd.com/digestive-disorders/exercise-curing-constipation-via-movement.

101 **use of poop-producing products:** Laura Dowart, "Excessive Laxative Use," Verywell Health, last updated August 12, 2023, https://www.verywellhealth.com/laxative-abuse-5219453.

101 **the small intestine is usually double:** Jill Seladi-Schulman, "What's the Length of Your Small and Large Intestines?," Healthline, last updated March 13, 2023, https://www.healthline.com/health/digestive-health/how-long-are-your-intestines#large-intestines.

102 **Fast food and other processed food:** Ida Judyta Malesza et al., "High-Fat, Western-Style Diet, Systemic Inflammation, and Gut Microbiota: A Narrative Review," *Cells* 10, no. 11 (2021): 3164, https://doi.org/10.3390/cells10113164.

102 **foods full of fiber:** "Eating, Diet, and Nutrition for Constipation," National Institute of Diabetes and Digestive and Kidney Diseases, last updated May 2018, https://www.niddk.nih.gov/health-information/digestive-diseases/constipation/eating-diet-nutrition.

102 **recommended grams of fiber:** Aelia Akbar and Apama P. Shreenath, "High Fiber Diet," StatPearls, last updated May 1, 2023, https://www.ncbi.nlm.nih.gov/books/NBK559033/.

102 **include water-filled foods:** Bethany Agusala, "25 Water-Rich Foods to Help You Stay Hydrated This Summer," *Prevention* (blog), UT Southwestern Medical Center, June 26, 2023, https://utswmed.org/medblog/hydrating-healthy-foods/.

102 **probiotics that can help:** Lisa Hayes, "What's the Deal with Probiotics?," Mayo Clinic Health System, September 15, 2021, https://www.mayoclinichealthsystem.org/hometown-health/speaking-of-health/whats-the-deal-with-probiotics.

103 **discomfort during bowel movements:** Bojana Galic, "Stomach Pain after Eating Spicy Food: Causes and Solutions," Livestrong, last updated August 14, 2023, https://www.livestrong.com/article/286244-stomach-pain-after-eating-spicy-food/.

103 **Urine is almost entirely water:** Neslihan Sarigul, Filiz Korkmaz, and İlhan Kurultak, "A New Artificial Urine Protocol to Better Imitate Human Urine," *Scientific Reports* 9, no. 1 (2019): 20159, https://doi.org/10.1038/s41598-019-56693-4.

103 **feces (poop) is 75 percent water:** Fermín Pérez-Guevara, Gurusamy Kutralam-Muniasamy, and V. C. Shruti, "Critical Review on Microplastics in Fecal Matter: Research Progress, Analytical Methods and Future Outlook," *Science of the Total Environment* 778 (2021): 146395, https://doi.org/10.1016/j.scitotenv.2021.146395.

103 **urine is a light-yellow color:** Samantha B. Kostelnik et al., "The Validity of Urine Color as a Hydration Biomarker within the General Adult Population and Athletes: A Systematic Review," *Journal of the American College of Nutrition* 40, no. 2 (2021): 172–79, https://doi.org/10.1080/07315724.2020.1750073.

103 **harder to pass:** Eric Blancaflor et al., "An IoT Design of a Dehydration Indicator System Based on Urine Color," in *2022 5th International Conference on Computing and Big Data* (IEEE, 2022), 118–22.

103 **drink approximately half a gallon:** Lawrence E. Armstrong and Evan C. Johnson, "Water Intake, Water Balance, and the Elusive Daily Water Requirement," *Nutrients* 10, no. 12 (2018): 1928, https://doi.org/10.3390/nu10121928.

103 **90 percent water:** Brianna Elliott, "19 Water-Rich Foods That Help You Stay Hydrated," Healthline, last updated February 7, 2023, https://www.healthline.com/nutrition/19-hydrating-foods.

103 **fiber, which helps with poop:** Ewa Stachowska et al., "Improvement of Bowel Movements among People with a Sedentary Lifestyle after Prebiotic Snack Supply—Preliminary Study," *Gastroenterology Review/Przegląd Gastroenterologiczny* 17, no. 1 (2022): 73–80, https://doi.org/10.5114/pg.2021.108985.

104 **excess water and the waste your kidneys filter:** "Urine and Urination," MedlinePlus, accessed January 9, 2024, https://medlineplus.gov/urineandurination.html.

104 **can hold up to 16 ounces:** "The Urinary Tract and How It Works." National Institute of Diabetes and Digestive and Kidney Diseases, February 28, 2023, https://www.niddk.nih.gov/health-information/urologic-diseases/urinary-tract-how-it-works.

104 **urine exits your body through the urethra:** Nicholas J. Lanzotti, Muhammad Ali Tariq, Srinivasa Rao Bolla, "Physiology, Bladder," StatPearls, last updated May 1, 2023, https://www.ncbi.nlm.nih.gov/books/NBK538533/.

104 **the urethral opening is usually:** "Urethra," National Cancer Institute SEER Training, Modules, accessed January 9, 2024, https://training.seer.cancer.gov/anatomy/urinary/components/urethra.html.

104 **seven times each day:** Chaunie Brusie and Daniel Yetman, "Does How Often You Pee Say Something about Your Health?," Healthline, last updated April 24, 2022, https://www.healthline.com/health/how-often-should-you-pee.

105 **more frequently or if:** Brusie and Yetman, "How Often You Pee."

105 **urobilin, a yellow chemical:** Rebekah Belasco et al., "The Effect of Hydration on Urine Color Objectively Evaluated in CIE L* a* b* Color Space," *Frontiers in Nutrition* 7 (2020): 576974, https://doi.org/10.3389/fnut.2020.576974.

105 **a darker shade:** "Dehydration," Cleveland Clinic, last updated June 5, 2023, https://my.clevelandclinic.org/health/treatments/9013-dehydration.

105 **Neon orange or yellow:** "Should I Be Worried about My Urine Color?" UnityPoint Health, accessed January 9, 2024, https://www.unitypoint.org/news-and-articles/should-i-be-worried-about-my-urine-color-unitypoint-health.

105 **Green could be:** "Urine Color," Mayo Clinic, January 10, 2023, https://www.mayoclinic.org/diseases-conditions/urine-color/symptoms-causes/syc-20367333.

105 **Pink can come:** Haley M. Sauder and Prashanth Rawla, "Beeturia," StatPearls, last updated May 22, 2023, https://www.ncbi.nlm.nih.gov/books/NBK537012/.

106 **Red urine could:** "Urine Color," Mayo Clinic.

106 **Dark orange-brown urine:** "Urine Color," Mayo Clinic.

106 **Black urine can:** Dilrai S. Kalsi et al., "Purple Urine Bag Syndrome: A Rare Spot Diagnosis," *Disease Markers* 2017 (2017), 9131872, https://doi.org/10.1155/2017/9131872.

106 **urine might stink:** Kalsi et al., "Purple Urine Bag Syndrome."

107 **a process called urinalysis:** "Urinalysis: What It Is, Purpose, Types and Results," Cleveland Clinic, last updated November 9, 2021, https://my.clevelandclinic.org/health/diagnostics/17893-urinalysis.

108 **1 in every 50 teenagers:** Blackwell Publishing, "One in 50 Teenagers Still Wet the Bed," Science Daily, May 18, 2006, https://www.sciencedaily.com/releases/2006/05/060517190502.htm.

108 **Drinking too much water:** Danielle Pacheco, "Drinking Water before Bed," Sleep Foundation, last updated December 7, 2023, https://www.sleepfoundation.org/nutrition/drinking-water-before-bed.

108 **even stress can affect:** Sarah Jenkins, "Ask the Doc: What Causes Bedwetting in Adults? (And How Can I Make It Stop?),"

National Association for Continence, accessed January 9, 2024, https://nafc.org/bhealth-blog/ask-the-expert-what-causes-bedwetting-in-adults-and-how-can-i-make-it-stop/.

108 **It can be hereditary:** A. von Gontard et al., "The Genetics of Enuresis," *Journal of Urology* 166, no. 6 (2001), 2438–43, https://doi.org/10.1097/00005392-200112000-00117.

108 **can be caused by constipation:** "Constipation," UCSF Department of Urology, accessed January 9, 2024, https://urology.ucsf.edu/patient-care/children/constipation.

108 **urinary tract infection (UTI for short):** "Urinary Tract Infection (UTI)," Mayo Clinic, September 14, 2022, https://www.mayoclinic.org/diseases-conditions/urinary-tract-infection/symptoms-causes/syc-20353447.

109 **UTIs are extremely common:** Kim Liner, "Urinary Tract Infections," Nurse-1-1, October 21, 2019, https://nurse-1-1.com/health/urinary-tract-infections/.

109 **Untreated UTIs can:** "Urinary Tract Infections," Sepsis Alliance, last updated June 7, 2023, https://www.sepsis.org/sepsisand/urinary-tract-infections.

109 **eliminating certain foods and beverages:** Mélanie Le Berre et al., "What Do We Really Know about the Role of Caffeine on Urinary Tract Symptoms? A Scoping Review on Caffeine Consumption and Lower Urinary Tract Symptoms in Adults," *Neurourology and Urodynamics* 39, no. 5 (2020): 1217–33, https://doi.org/10.1002/nau.24344.

110 **kidney stones are on the rise:** Katie Camero, "Kidney Stones Are Rising among Children and Teens, Especially Girls, Research Shows," NBC News, July 8, 2023, https://www.nbcnews.com/health/kids

-health/kidney-stones-nephrolithiasis-kids
-teens-girls-rcna91431.

110 **solid masses called kidney stones:** "Kidney Stones," National Institute of Diabetes and Digestive and Kidney Diseases, accessed January 9, 2024, https://www.niddk.nih .gov/health-information/urologic-diseases /kidney-stones.

110 **bigger stones cannot pass:** Kelcy Higa et al., "The Case of an Obstructed Stone at the Distal Urethra," *Cureus* 9, no. 12 (2017): c1974, https://doi.org/10.7759/cureus.1974.

110 **water can help:** "6 Easy Ways to Prevent Kidney Stones," National Kidney Foundation, accessed January 9, 2024, https://www.kidney.org/atoz /content/kidneystones_prevent#don-t -underestimate-your-sweat.

110 **up to twenty-five times each day:** "Symptoms and Causes of Gas in the Digestive Tract," National Institute of Diabetes and Digestive and Kidney Diseases, last updated June 2021, https:// www.niddk.nih.gov/health-information /digestive-diseases/gas-digestive-tract /symptoms-causes.

111 **swallowing excess air:** Vikram Rangan et al., "Belching: Pathogenesis, Clinical Characteristics, and Treatment Strategies," *Journal of Clinical Gastroenterology* 56, no. 1 (2022): 36–40, https://doi.org /10.1097/MCG.0000000000001631.

111 **Stinky farts, however:** Diane Abraczinskas, "Overview of Intestinal Gas and Bloating," MediLib UpToDate, December 2023, https://medilib.ir/uptodate/show/2607.

111 **common high-gas culprits:** Rena Goldman, "10 Foods That Cause Gas," Healthline, last updated February 16, 2023, https://www .healthline.com/health/foods-that-cause -gas.

111 **carbonated drinks like soda:** "Belching, Bloating, and Flatulence Overview,"

American College of Gastroenterology, last updated January 2022, https://gi.org /topics/belching-bloating-and-flatulence/.

111 **symptom of which is heartburn:** Maartje Singendonk et al., "Prevalence of Gastroesophageal Reflux Disease Symptoms in Infants and Children: A Systematic Review," *Journal of Pediatric Gastroenterology and Nutrition* 68, no. 6 (2019): 811–17, https://doi.org/10.1097 /MPG.0000000000002280

111 **if there's post-eating pain:** "Acid Reflux, Heartburn, and GERD: What's the Difference?," NIH MedlinePlus Magazine, January 24, 2020, https://magazine .medlineplus.gov/article/acid-reflux -heartburn-and-gerd-whats-the-difference.

111 **suffer from no-burp syndrome:** "This Is What Happens When You Cannot Burp, Ever," Columbia University Irving Medical Center, June 9, 2022, https://www.cuimc .columbia.edu/news/what-happens-when -you-cannot-burp-ever.

111 **unable to fart:** Isadora Baum, "The Health Benefits of Farting," *Men's Health*, September 20, 2020, https://www.mens health.com/health/a33983694/farting -healthy-benefits/.

112 **reasons people become bloated:** "Bloating," familydoctor.org, last updated June 2023, https://familydoctor.org/condition/bloating/.

112 **exercise, stomach massage:** Min-Ja Lee, "13 Yoga Poses to Relieve Gas and Bloating," *Health*, last updated July 12, 2023, https:// www.health.com/fitness/beat-bloat-with -yoga.

113 **impossible to comfortably digest:** Peter Jaret, "Bloating 101: Why You Feel Bloated," WebMD, last updated April 15, 2022, https://www.webmd.com/digestive -disorders/features/bloated-bloating.

113 **gluten might not be great for your body:** "Gluten Intolerance," Cleveland

Clinic, last updated June 30, 2021, https://my.clevelandclinic.org/health /diseases/21622-gluten-intolerance.

114 1 out of every 6: Kaitlin E. Occhipinti and James W. Smith, "Irritable Bowel Syndrome: A Review and Update," *Clinics in Colon and Rectal Surgery* 25, no. 1 (2012): 46–52, https://doi.org/10.1055/s -0032-1301759.

114 feeling worse after eating: "Diagnosis of Irritable Bowel Syndrome," National Institute of Diabetes and Digestive and Kidney Diseases, last updated November 2017, https://www.niddk.nih.gov/health -information/digestive-diseases/irritable -bowel-syndrome/diagnosis.

114 cause intestinal inflammation: Gwo-Tzer Ho et al., "Resolution of Inflammation and Gut Repair in IBD: Translational Steps Towards Complete Mucosal Healing," *Inflammatory Bowel Diseases* 26, no. 8 (2020): 1131–43, https://doi.org/10.1093/ ibd/izaa045.

114 including Crohn's disease: Gian Paolo Caviglia et al., "Epidemiology of Inflammatory Bowel Diseases: A Population Study in a Healthcare District of North-West Italy." *Journal of Clinical Medicine* 12, no. 2 (2023): 641, https://doi .org/10.3390/jcm12020641.

114 IBD symptoms can: Marc Fakhoury et al., "Inflammatory Bowel Disease: Clinical Aspects and Treatments," *Journal of Inflammation Research* 23, no. 7 (2014): 113–20, https://doi.org/10.2147/jir.s65979.

114 celiac disease is: "What Is Celiac Disease?," Celiac Disease Foundation, accessed January 9, 2024, https://celiac.org/about -celiac-disease/what-is-celiac-disease/.

Genitalia (Penises & Vulvas)

118 with different shapes: "Episode 1: Meet Your Vagina and Vulva," Planned Parenthood, YouTube video, October 4, 2017, https://www.youtube.com /watch?v=SiOE7DsCJIM&t=1s.

118 three main functions: John D. Nguyen and Hieu Duong, "Anatomy, Abdomen and Pelvis: Female External Genitalia," StatPearls, last updated July 25, 2022, https://www.ncbi.nlm.nih.gov/books /NBK547703.

118 "normal" penis or vulva: Nguyen and Duong, "Anatomy, Abdomen and Pelvis."

118 inside the scrotum: "Gonads," National Cancer Institute SEER Training Modules, accessed January 9, 2024, https://training .seer.cancer.gov/anatomy/endocrine/glands /gonads.html.

120 each side of the uterus: Rodolfo Rey, Nathalie Josso, and Chrystèle Racine, "Sexual Differentiation," Endotext, last updated May 27, 2020, https://www.ncbi .nlm.nih.gov/books/NBK279001/.

120 testicles and ovaries both develop: Owuraku A. Titi-Lartey and Yusuf S. Khan, "Embryology, Testicle," StatPearls, last updated April 24, 2023, https://www.ncbi .nlm.nih.gov/books/NBK557763.

120 activate at puberty: Margaret R. Bell, "Comparing Postnatal Development of Gonadal Hormones and Associated Social Behaviors in Rats, Mice, and Humans," *Endocrinology* 159, no. 7 (2018): 2596–613, https://doi.org/10.1210/en.2018-00220.

120 producing the same key hormones: "Reproductive Hormones," Endocrine Society, January 24, 2022, https://www .endocrine.org/patient-engagement /endocrine-library/hormones-and -endocrine-function/reproductive -hormones.

121 level of skin darkening: Carla Sebastián- Enesco and Gün R. Semin, "The Brightness Dimension as a Marker of Gender across Cultures and Age," *Psychological*

Research/Psychologische Forschung 84, no. 8 (2020): 2375–84, https://doi.org /10.1007/s00426-019-01213-2.

121 **if new colorations are paired:** Christine Case-Lo and Kristeen Cherney, "What Causes Skin Discoloration?," Healthline, last updated August 3, 2023, https://www .healthline.com/health/discolored-skin -patches.

121 **other unpleasant sensation:** "Vaginal Discharge," Cleveland Clinic, last updated July 22, 2022, https://my.clevelandclinic .org/health/symptoms/4719-vaginal -discharge.

121 **Itchy genitalia could:** "Vaginitis," MedlinePlus, accessed January 9, 2024, https://medlineplus.gov/vaginitis.html.

121 **genital psoriasis or eczema:** Linda Rath, "Genital Psoriasis: Signs and Symptoms to Look For," WebMD, last updated September 14, 2023, https://www.webmd .com/skin-problems-and-treatments /psoriasis/genital-psoriasis-signs -symptoms.

122 **your personal *eau de you*:** Ginger Wojcik, "Molasses to Pennies: All the Smells a Healthy Vagina Can Be," Healthline, last updated February 8, 2023, https://www .healthline.com/health/womens-health /vagina-smells#5.-Skunky-like-BO-or -a-smoked-herbal,-earthy-scent.

122 **altered for the worse:** Wojcik, "Molasses to Pennies."

123 **Jock itch can also:** Rachel Nall, "Does Jock Itch Have an Odor?," Healthline, last updated April 7, 2023, https://www .healthline.com/health/jock-itch-smell.

124 **penile enlargement or labiaplasty:** Bruce M. King, "Average-Size Erect Penis: Fiction, Fact, and the Need for Counseling," *Journal of Sex and Marital Therapy* 47, no. 1 (2021): 80–89, https://doi.org/10.1080/0092623x .2020.1787279.

124 **pressure for "perfection":** Margo Mullinax et al., "In Their Own Words: A Qualitative Content Analysis of Women's and Men's Preferences for Women's Genitals," *Sex Education* 15, no. 4 (2015): 421–36, https:// doi.org/10.1080/14681811.2015.1031884.

124 **"average" genitalia size:** Gemma Sharp et al., "Beyond Motivations: A Qualitative Pilot Exploration of Women's Experiences Prior to Labiaplasty," *Aesthetic Surgery Journal* 43, no. 9 (2023): 994–1001, https://doi .org/10.1093/asj/sjad105.

125 **study one ethnicity:** A. Kreklau et al., "Measurements of a 'Normal Vulva' in Women Aged 15–84: A Cross-Sectional Prospective Single-Centre Study," *BJOG: An International Journal of Obstetrics and Gynaecology* 125, no. 13 (2018): 1656–61, https://doi.org/10.1111/1471-0528.15387.

125 **leave out specific demographics:** Aşkı Ellibeş Kaya et al., "Do External Female Genital Measurements Affect Genital Perception and Sexual Function and Orgasm?," *Türk Jinekoloji Ve Obstetrik Derneği Dergisi* 17, no. 3 (2020) 175–81, https://doi.org/10.4274/tjod.galenos .2020.89896.

125 **perineum stretches to help:** "Perineum," Cleveland Clinic, October 26, 2022, https://my.clevelandclinic.org/health /body/24381-perineum.

126 **Smegma is a whitish:** Kimberly Holland, "Everything You Should Know about Smegma," Healthline, last updated February 13, 2023, https://www.healthline .com/health/smegma.

126 **break up penile adhesions:** "Penile Adhesions," Children's Hospital of Philadelphia, accessed January 9, 2024, https://www.chop.edu/conditions -diseases/penile-adhesions.

127 **Lumps or bumps:** Kristeen Cherney, "How to Identify and Treat an Ingrown Hair

Cyst," Healthline, last updated May 19, 2023, https://www.healthline.com/health/beauty-skin-care/ingrown-hair-cyst.

127 **Two scary-looking (at first):** M. Yeo, "10 Causes of Abnormal Vaginal Lumps and Bumps," DTAP Medical Clinic, September 25, 2018, https://www.dtapclinic.com/articles/10-causes-of-abnormal-vaginal-lumps-and-bumps/

127 **bumps could be a sign:** Frank DiVincenzo, "Genital Warts vs. Herpes: Difference, Causes and Treatments," K Health, last updated May 6, 2022, https://khealth.com/learn/herpes/vs-genital-warts.

127 **human papillomavirus (HPV):** "Anal Warts," Cleveland Clinic, last updated September 2, 2022, https://my.clevelandclinic.org/health/diseases/24097-anal-warts.

127 **skin-to-skin contact with:** Rayleen M. Lewis et al., "Prevalence of Genital Human Papillomavirus among Sexually Experienced Males and Females Aged 14–59 Years, United States, 2013–2014," *Journal of Infectious Diseases* 217, no. 6 (2018): 869–77, https://doi.org/10.1093/infdis/jix655.

127 **eligible for the HPV vaccine:** "HPV Vaccine Information for Young Women," Centers for Disease Control and Prevention, last updated April 18, 2022, https://www.cdc.gov/std/hpv/stdfact-hpv-vaccine-young-women.htm.

127 **additional HPV complications:** "Genital Warts," Mayo Clinic, last updated June 30, 2023, https://www.mayoclinic.org/diseases-conditions/genital-warts/diagnosis-treatment/drc-20355240.

127 **herpes simplex virus 2:** "Herpes Simplex Virus," World Health Organization, April 5, 2023, https://www.who.int/news-room/fact-sheets/detail/herpes-simplex-virus.

127 **more than 10 percent:** "Genital Herpes—CDC Detailed Fact Sheet," Centers for Disease Control and Prevention, last updated July 22, 2021, https://www.cdc.gov/std/herpes/stdfact-herpes-detailed.htm.

128 **herpes simplex virus 1:** "Cold Sores," Cleveland Clinic, last updated April 27, 2023, https://my.clevelandclinic.org/health/diseases/21136-cold-sores.

128 **See your doctor for diagnosis:** "Herpes Simplex Virus," World Health Organization.

128 **medication can help:** "Sexually Transmitted Diseases (STDs)," Mayo Clinic, last updated September 8, 2023, https://www.mayoclinic.org/diseases-conditions/sexually-transmitted-diseases-stds/diagnosis-treatment/drc-20351246.

128 *never* **pop bumps:** "Sexually Transmitted Disease (STD) Symptoms," Mayo Clinic, last updated May 5, 2022, https://www.mayoclinic.org/diseases-conditions/sexually-transmitted-diseases-stds/in-depth/std-symptoms/art-20047081.

128 **the anus is actually:** "Your Digestive System," University of Michigan Health, accessed January 9, 2024, https://www.uofmhealth.org/conditions-treatments/digestive-and-liver-health/your-digestive-system.

128 **The visible parts:** "Overview of the Male Anatomy," Johns Hopkins Medicine, accessed January 9, 2024, https://www.hopkinsmedicine.org/health/wellness-and-prevention/overview-of-the-male-anatomy.

128 **While always cylindrical:** Peter Sam and Chad A. LaGrange, "Anatomy, Abdomen and Pelvis, Penis," StatPearls, last updated on July 24, 2023, https://www.ncbi.nlm.nih.gov/books/NBK482236/.

129 **The rounded head:** "Glans Penis," Healthline, last updated July 5, 2023, https://www.healthline.com/human-body-maps/glans-penis#1.

129 **The rounded ridge:** Sam and LaGrange, "Anatomy, Abdomen and Pelvis, Penis."

129 **different hygiene routines:** Beth Sissons, "What to Know about Circumcised and Uncircumcised Penises," MedicalNewsToday, last updated June 26, 2023, https://www.medicalnewstoday.com/articles/325713.

129 **foreskin protects the glans:** "Foreskin," Cleveland Clinic, last updated May 31, 2022, https://my.clevelandclinic.org/health/body/23175-foreskin.

129 **procedure called circumcision:** "Circumcision (Male)," Mayo Clinic," last updated March 22, 2022, https://www.mayoclinic.org/tests-procedures/circumcision/about/pac-20393550.

129 **religious or cultural reasons:** "Circumcision," Cleveland Clinic, last updated January 23, 2021, https://my.clevelandclinic.org/health/treatments/16194-circumcision.

129 **Vulvas also have a fold:** Adrienne Santos-Longhurst, "Everything You Should Know about Your Clitoral Hood," Healthline, last updated February 9, 2023, https://www.healthline.com/health/womens-health/clitoral-hood

130 **The raised ridge:** "Penis Frenulum," Cleveland Clinic, last updated July 25, 2022, https://my.clevelandclinic.org/health/body/23533-penis-frenulum.

130 **powerful erogenous zone:** Hayley Krischer, "7 Awesome Erogenous Zones," WebMD, October 13, 2015, https://www.webmd.com/sex-relationships/features/7-awesome-erogenous-zones.

130 **A slit in the penis:** "Glans Penis," Healthline.

130 **urine and semen exit:** "The Urinary Tract System," Urology Care Foundation, accessed January 9, 2024, https://www.urologyhealth.org/urology-a-z/the-urinary-tract-system.

130 **This is known as hypospadias:** Alvaro E. Donaire and Magda D. Mendez, "Hypospadias," StatPearls, last updated July 31, 2023, https://www.ncbi.nlm.nih.gov/books/NBK482122.

131 **called pearly penile papules:** Adam S. Aldahan, Tara K. Brah, and Keyvan Nouri, "Diagnosis and Management of Pearly Penile Papules," *American Journal of Men's Health* 12, no. 3 (2018): 624–27, https://doi.org/10.1177/1557988316654138.

131 **(pull back) their foreskin:** "Care for an Uncircumcised Penis," Healthy Children, last updated June 19, 2017, https://www.healthychildren.org/English/ages-stages/baby/bathing-skin-care/Pages/Care-for-an-Uncircumcised-Penis.aspx.

131 **is called phimosis:** "Phimosis," Nationwide Children's, accessed January 9, 2024, https://www.nationwidechildrens.org/conditions/phimosis.

132 **forcibly pulling the foreskin:** James Roland, "Everything You Should Know about Phimosis," Healthline, last updated September 29, 2018, https://www.healthline.com/health/mens-health/phimosis.

132 **is called paraphimosis:** Bradley N. Bragg, Erwin L. Kong, and Stephen W. Leslie, "Paraphimosis," StatPearls, last updated on May 30, 2023, https://www.ncbi.nlm.nih.gov/books/NBK459233.

132 **foreskin remains retracted:** Bragg, Kong, and Leslie, "Paraphimosis."

132 **foreskin can become inflamed:** Adrienne Santos-Longhurst. "What to Know about Balanitis," Healthline, March 20, 2023, https://www.healthline.com/health/balanitis.

132 **called a penile adhesion:** James Roland, "Penile Adhesions," Healthline, last updated December 7, 2018. https://www.healthline.com/health/penile-adhesion.

133 **Zipper teeth can:** Stephen W. Leslie, Hussain Sajjad, and Roger S. Taylor, "Penile Zipper and Ring Injuries," StatPearls, last updated May 30, 2023, https://www.ncbi.nlm.nih.gov/books/NBK441886/.

133 **can get urinary tract infections:** Robert H. Shmerling, "Urinary Tract Infection in Men," *Harvard Health*, December 5, 2022, https://www.health.harvard.edu/a_to_z/urinary-tract-infection-in-men-a-to-z.

133 **Discharge is any liquid:** "Vaginal Discharge," Mayo Clinic, April 25, 2023, https://www.mayoclinic.org/symptoms/vaginal-discharge/basics/definition/sym-20050825.

133 **inflammation or an infection:** Donna Christiano, "Is Male Discharge Normal?," Healthline, last updated April 17, 2023, https://www.healthline.com/health/male-discharge-normal.

134 **fungal infection around the genitalia:** Barbara Kean, "What Is Jock Itch? Symptoms, Causes, Diagnosis, Treatment, and Prevention," Everyday Health, February 25, 2023, https://www.everydayhealth.com/jock-itch/.

134 **scrotum contains the testicles:** "Testicles," Cleveland Clinic, August 9, 2022, https://my.clevelandclinic.org/health/body/23964-testicles.

134 **born with an undescended testicle:** Stephen W. Leslie, Hussain Sajjad, and Carlos A. Villanueva, "Cryptorchidism," StatPearls, last updated June 5, 2023, https://www.ncbi.nlm.nih.gov/books/NBK470270.

134 **developing testicular cancer:** "Risk Factors for Testicular Cancer," American Cancer Society, last updated May 17, 2018, https://www.cancer.org/cancer/types/testicular-cancer/causes-risks-prevention/risk-factors.html.

134 **Sometimes testicles are retractile:** Piyush K. Agarwal, Mireya Diaz, and Jack S. Elder, "Retractile Testis—Is It Really a Normal Variant?," *Journal of Urology* 175, no. 4 (2006): 1496–99, https://doi.org/10.1016/S0022-5347(05)00674-9.

135 **if you have testicular pain:** "Testicular Trauma," Cleveland Clinic, April 10, 2022, https://my.clevelandclinic.org/health/diseases/22814-testicular-trauma.

135 **like testicular torsion:** "Testicular Torsion," Mayo Clinic, February 24, 2022, https://www.mayoclinic.org/diseases-conditions/testicular-torsion/symptoms-causes/syc-20378270.

135 **growth during puberty:** "Testicular Torsion: Signs, Causes, and What to Do," Children's Health, accessed January 9, 2024, https://www.childrens.com/health-wellness/testicular-torsion-signs-causes-what-to-do.

135 **permanent testicular damage:** "Testicular Failure," MedlinePlus Medical Encyclopedia, last updated May 12, 2023, https://medlineplus.gov/ency/article/000395.htm.

135 **Testicular cancer is the most:** Jee Soo Park et al., "Recent Global Trends in Testicular Cancer Incidence and Mortality," *Medicine* (Baltimore) 97 (37): e12390, https://doi.org/10.1097/md.0000000000012390.

135 **ideally in the shower:** "Self-Check for Testicular Cancer," Testicular Cancer Foundation, accessed January 9, 2024, https://www.testicularcancer.org/testicular-self-exam/.

136 **one testicle is larger:** Bethany Cadman, "Is It Normal to Have Differently Sized Testicles?," MedicalNewsToday, last updated July 24, 2023, https://www.medicalnewstoday.com/articles/321234.

136 **that's the epididymis:** S. Marchiani et al., "Epididymal Sperm Transport and Fertilization," *Endocrinology of the Testis and Male Reproduction* 1 (2017): 457–78, https://doi.org/10.1007/978-3-319 -29456-8_14-1.

136 **roll the testicle:** "Self-Check for Testicular Cancer," Testicular Cancer Foundation.

137 **any new developments:** "How to Perform a Testicular Self-Exam: Advice from Urologist Nirmish Singla," Johns Hopkins Medicine, May 9, 2022, https://www .hopkinsmedicine.org/health/conditions -and-diseases/testicular-cancer/how-to -perform-a-testicular-selfexam-advice -from-urologist-nirmish-singla.

137 **called a varicocele:** "Varicocele," Mayo Clinic, March 3, 2022, https://www .mayoclinic.org/diseases-conditions /varicocele/symptom.

137 **caught and treated early:** Testicular Cancer Society, accessed January 9, 2024, https://testicularcancersociety.org.

137 **The penis has two states:** Kimberly Holland, "Everything You Need to Know about a Flaccid Penis," Healthline, October 10, 2019, https://www.healthline .com/health/mens-health/flaccid-penis.

138 **Erections occur for:** Robert C. Dean and Tom F. Lue, "Physiology of Penile Erection and Pathophysiology of Erectile Dysfunction," *Urologic Clinics of North America* 32, no. 4 (2005): 379–95, https:// doi.org/10.1016/j.ucl.2005.08.007.

139 **a minute or two to half an hour:** "Premature Ejaculation: Overview," InformedHealth.org, September 12, 2019. https://www.ncbi.nlm.nih.gov/books /NBK547548/.

139 **ignored long enough:** Pranau K. Panchatsharam, Justin Durland, and Patrick M. Zito, "Physiology, Erection," StatPearls, last updated May 1, 2023, https://www.ncbi.nlm.nih.gov/books /NBK513278/.

139 **"coming" or "climaxing":** "Orgasms," Planned Parenthood, accessed January 9, 2024, https://www.plannedparenthood .org/learn/sex-pleasure-and-sexual -dysfunction/sex-and-pleasure/orgasms.

140 **"ejected" out of the tip:** Yiji Suh et al., "Etiologic Classification, Evaluation, and Management of Hematospermia," *Translational Andrology and Urology* 6, no. 5 (2017): 959–72, https://doi .org/10.21037/tau.2017.06.01.

140 **process is called ejaculation:** Adrienne Santos-Longhurst, "What's the Difference between Semen and Sperm? And 12 Other FAQs," Healthline, August 31, 2020, https://www.healthline.com/health /semen-vs-sperm#difference.

140 **Semen contains sperm:** "Conception: How It Works," UCSF Health, accessed January 9, 2024, https://www.ucsfhealth .org/education/conception-how-it-works.

140 **less than 1 teaspoon:** Zawn Villines, "What to Know about Ejaculate Volume and Distance," MedicalNewsToday, last updated March 31, 2023, https://www .medicalnewstoday.com/articles/how-far -can-a-man-shoot#averages.

140 **back to its flaccid state:** Panchatsharam, Durland, and Zito, "Physiology, Erection."

140 **ejaculate without orgasm:** Marisa Gray et al., "Contemporary Management of Ejaculatory Dysfunction," *Translational Andrology and Urology* 7, no. 4 (2018): 686–702, https://doi.org/10.21037 /tau.2018.06.20.

140 **no ejaculated semen:** "Dry Orgasm," Mayo Clinic, November 30, 2022, https://www .mayoclinic.org/symptoms/dry-orgasm /basics/causes/sym-20050906.

141 **doesn't contain sperm:** Scaccia, Annamarya, "Can You Get Pregnant from Pre-Cum? What to Expect," Healthline, last updated September 20, 2022.

141 **can also transmit:** S. Nicole Lane, "What Is Precum?," Verywell Health, last updated May 8, 2023, https://www.verywellhealth.com/what-is-precum-5085078.

141 **as "nocturnal emissions":** Annamarya Scaccia, "Can Vagina Owners Have Wet Dreams, Too? And Other Questions Answered," Healthline, last updated September 8, 2023, https://www.healthline.com/health/healthy-sex/wet-dreams.

141 **don't have the organs to produce semen:** Scaccia, "Can Vagina Owners Have Wet Dreams, Too?"

141 **cause of penile fractures:** Md. Jawaid Rahman et al., "Penile Manipulation: The Most Common Etiology of Penile Fracture at Our Tertiary Care Center." *Journal of Family Medicine and Primary Care* 5, no. 2 (2016): 471–73, https://doi.org/10.4103/2249-4863.192347.

141 **happen during other:** Kyle C. Diaz and Heather Cronovich, "Penis Fracture," StatPearls, last updated July 29, 2022, https://www.ncbi.nlm.nih.gov/books/NBK551618/.

142 **Signs of a fractured penis:** "Is It Possible to Fracture Your Penis? [answer from Matthew J. Ziegelmann, MD]," Mayo Clinic, July 29, 2022, https://www.mayoclinic.org/healthy-lifestyle/sexual-health/expert-answers/penis-fracture/faq-20058154.

142 **is called priapism:** Michael Silberman et al., "Priapism," StatPearls, last updated May 30, 2023, https://www.ncbi.nlm.nih.gov/books/NBK459178.

142 **can cause permanent damage:** Silberman et al., "Priapism."

142 **the hormone testosterone surging:** "Testosterone," You and Your Hormones from the Society for Endocrinology, last updated December 2020, https://www.yourhormones.info/hormones/testosterone/.

142 **known as erectile dysfunction or impotence:** Giulia Rastrelli and Mario Maggi, "Erectile Dysfunction in Fit and Healthy Young Men: Psychological or Pathological?," *Translational Andrology and Urology* 6, no. 1 (2017): 79–90, https://doi.org/10.21037/tau.2016.09.06.

143 **stops being stimulated:** Neel Duggal, "Guide to Epididymal Hypertension (Blue Balls)," Healthline, last updated October 14, 2021, https://www.healthline.com/health/mens-health/blue-balls.

143 **medical name, epididymal hypertension:** Beth Sissons, "Is Blue Balls a Real Condition?" MedicalNewsToday, last updated October 17, 2023, https://www.medicalnewstoday.com/articles/324870.

143 **some say "blue bean":** Melissa Persensky, "'Blue Balls': Facts and Fiction," *Health Essentials* (blog), Cleveland Clinic, January 18, 2023, https://health.clevelandclinic.org/blue-balls/.

143 **collection of external (visible) genitalia:** "What Are the Parts of the Female Sexual Anatomy?," Planned Parenthood, accessed January 9, 2024, https://www.plannedparenthood.org/learn/health-and-wellness/sexual-and-reproductive-anatomy/what-are-parts-female-sexual-anatomy.

144 **slightly longer than the right:** A. Kreklau et al., "Measurements of a 'Normal Vulva' in Women Aged 15–84: A Cross-Sectional Prospective Single-Centre Study," *BJOG: An International Journal of Obstetrics and Gynaecology* 125, no. 13 (2018): 1656–61, https://doi.org/10.1111/1471-0528.15387.

144 **Bartholin's cyst can form:** "Bartholin's Cyst," Mayo Clinic, April 30, 2022, https://www.mayoclinic.org/diseases-conditions/bartholin-cyst/symptoms-causes/syc-20369976.

145 **the bean-like tip:** "Clitoris," Cleveland Clinic, last updated April 25, 2022, https://my.clevelandclinic.org/health/body/22823-clitoris.

145 **skin fold covers the tip:** Adrienne Santos-Longhurst, "Everything You Should Know about Your Clitoral Hood," Healthline, last updated February 9, 2023, https://www.healthline.com/health/womens-health/clitoral-hood.

145 **Just below the clitoral glans:** "How Many Holes Does a Female Body Have Down There?," Planned Parenthood, October 28, 2019, https://www.plannedparenthood.org/blog/help-i-know-alot-about-sex-and-everything-but-i-dont-know-anything-about-what-holes-are-for-what-i-dont-even-know-how-many-are-down-there-please-help.

145 **the opening to the vagina:** "Are My Vulva and Vagina Normal?," Planned Parenthood, accessed January 9, 2024, https://www.plannedparenthood.org/learn/teens/puberty/my-vulva-and-vagina-normal.

146 **about the same as:** Alexandra Benisek, "Anatomy, Function, Care, and Conditions of the Clitoris," WebMD, November 8, 2022, https://www.webmd.com/women/anatomy-function-care-conditions-clitoris.

146 **Stimulating the clitoris:** Jennifer Chesak and Gabrielle Kassel, "The Ultimate Guide to Clitoral Stimulation," Healthline, last updated February 28, 2023, https://www.healthline.com/health/healthy-sex/clitoris.

146 **some fluid can be released:** Chesak and Kassel, "The Ultimate Guide."

146 **it isn't urine:** Félix D. Rodríguez et al., "Female Ejaculation: An Update on Anatomy, History, and Controversies," *Clinical Anatomy* 34, no. 1 (2021): 103–107, https://doi.org/10.1002/ca.23654.

146 **vagina is a tunnel-shaped organ:** Benisek, "Anatomy, Function, Care."

147 **all vaginas have in common:** Joann M. Gold and Isha Shrimanker, "Physiology, Vaginal," StatPearls, last updated July 24, 2023, https://www.ncbi.nlm.nih.gov/books/NBK545147.

147 **vagina is the "birth canal":** "birth canal," in Merriam-Webster Dictionary, accessed January 8, 2024, https://www.merriam-webster.com/dictionary/birth%20canal.

147 **It's not uncommon for:** Leslie A. Sadownik, "Etiology, Diagnosis, and Clinical Management of Vulvodynia," *International Journal of Women's Health* 6 (2014): 437–49, https://doi.org/10.2147/IJWH.S37660.

147 **this kind of pain:** "Vaginal Pain: Causes and How to Treat It," MedicalNewsToday, May 23, 2023, https://www.medicalnewstoday.com/articles/326977.

148 **conditions like vulvodynia:** Camille A. Clare and John Yeh, "Vulvodynia in Adolescence: Childhood Vulvar Pain Syndromes," *Journal of Pediatric and Adolescent Gynecology* 24, no. 3 (2011): 110–15, https://doi.org/10.1016/j.jpag.2010.08.009.

148 **including physical therapy:** Stephanie A. Prendergast, "Pelvic Floor Physical Therapy for Vulvodynia," *Obstetrics and Gynecology Clinics of North America* 44, no. 3 (2017): 509–22, https://doi.org/10.1016/j.ogc.2017.05.006.

148 **right before or during their period:** Dani Blum, "Why Do I Feel Sick Before My Period?," *New York Times*, May 3, 2022, https://www.nytimes.com/2022/05/03/well/sick-before-period-symptoms.html.

148 **starts a new cycle:** Lisa B. Hurwitz et al., "'When You're a Baby You Don't Have Puberty': Understanding of Puberty and Human Reproduction in Late Childhood and Early Adolescence," *Journal of Early Adolescence* 37, no. 7 (2017): 925–47, https://doi.org/10.1177/0272431616642323.

148 **process called ovulation:** Julie E. Holesh, Autumn N. Bass, and Megan Lord, "Physiology, Ovulation," StatPearls, last updated May 1, 2023, https://www.ncbi.nlm.nih.gov/books/NBK441996.

148 **called the uterine lining:** "The Menstrual Cycle: An Overview," Stanford Medicine Children's Health, accessed January 9, 2024, https://www.stanfordchildrens.org/en/topic/default?id=menstrual-cycle-an-overview-85-P00553.

149 **muscles in the uterus contract:** "Menstruation," MedlinePlus, May 22, 2017, https://medlineplus.gov/menstruation.html.

149 **called menstrual blood:** "Menstruation," MedlinePlus.

149 **range in color:** Ashley Marcin and Adrienne Santos-Longhurst, "Black, Brown, Bright Red, and More: What Does Each Period Blood Color Mean?," Healthline, last updated March 8, 2023, https://www.healthline.com/health/period-blood.

149 **releases about 5 tablespoons:** William H. Parker, "Menstrual Disorders," HealthyWomen, September 16, 2009, https://www.healthywomen.org/condition/menstrual-disorders.

149 **menstrual blood contains clots:** Donna Christiano, "What Causes Menstrual Clots and Are My Clots Normal?," Healthline, last updated April 18, 2023, https://www.healthline.com/health/womens-health/menstrual-clots.

149 **takes three to seven days:** "Menstrual Cycle," Better Health Channel, Victoria State Government Department of Health, accessed January 9, 2024, https://www.betterhealth.vic.gov.au/health/conditionsandtreatments/menstrual-cycle.

149 **uterus regrows a new lining:** "Menstrual Cycle: An Overview," Johns Hopkins Medicine, accessed January 9, 2024, https://www.hopkinsmedicine.org/health/wellness-and-prevention/menstrual-cycle-an-overview.

149 **fluctuations are normal:** Rachel Nall, "Why Is My Period So Light?," MedicalNewsToday, last updated April 14, 2023, https://www.medicalnewstoday.com/articles/322935.

150 **a heavier-than-normal period:** "Heavy Menstrual Bleeding," Mayo Clinic, August 30, 2023, https://www.mayoclinic.org/diseases-conditions/menorrhagia/symptoms-causes/syc-20352829.

150 **Menorrhagia is a symptom:** "Heavy Menstrual Bleeding," Centers for Disease Control and Prevention, last updated June 23, 2023, https://www.cdc.gov/ncbddd/blooddisorders/women/menorrhagia.html.

150 **first few years of menstruating:** "Irregular Periods," NHS Inform, last updated February 28, 2023, https://www.nhsinform.scot/healthy-living/womens-health/girls-and-young-women-puberty-to-around-25/periods-and-menstrual-health/irregular-periods.

150 **anyone could miss a period:** Cassandra Holloway, "Yes, Weight Loss Can Impact Your Menstrual Cycle," *Health Essentials* (blog), Cleveland Clinic, April 7, 2023, https://health.clevelandclinic.org/can-weight-loss-affect-your-period.

151 **and every few days after:** "How Many Pregnancy Tests Should You Take?," Clearblue, last updated October 13, 2023,

https://www.clearblue.com/am-i-pregnant/how-many-pregnancy-tests-should-i-take.

151 **2,280 days, or over six years:** "The True Cost of Your Period," *Pandia Health* (blog), last updated May 7, 2021, https://www.pandiahealth.com/blog/the-true-cost-of-your-period/.

151 **450 menstrual periods:** L. R. H. Americas, "Menstrual Health: A Neglected Public Health Problem," *Lancet Regional Health—Americas* 15 (2022): 100399, doi: 10.1016/j.lana.2022.100399.

151 **issue called secondary amenorrhea:** "Amenorrhea," Mayo Clinic, last updated February 9, 2023, https://www.mayoclinic.org/diseases-conditions/amenorrhea/symptoms-causes/syc-20369299.

151 **more serious problem, such as:** "Amenorrhea," Mayo Clinic.

151 **birth control prevents:** Nall, "Why Is My Period So Light?"

152 **on a regular basis:** "Heavy and Abnormal Periods," American College of Obstetricians and Gynecologists, last updated August 2022, https://www.acog.org/womens-health/faqs/heavy-and-abnormal-periods.

152 **Formally known as dysmenorrhea:** Liwen Wang et al., "Prevalence and Risk Factors of Primary Dysmenorrhea in Students: A Meta-Analysis," *Value in Health* 25, no. 10 (2022): 1678–84, https://doi.org/10.1016/j.jval.2022.03.023.

152 **most painful on the heaviest day:** Mariagiulia Bernardi et al., "Dysmenorrhea and Related Disorders," *F1000Research* 6 (2017): 1645, https://doi.org/10.12688/f1000research.11682.1.

153 **Exercise also releases endorphins:** Narges Motahari-Tabari, Marjan Ahmad Shirvani, and Abbas Alipour, "Comparison of the Effect of Stretching Exercises and Mefenamic Acid on the Reduction of Pain and Menstruation Characteristics in Primary Dysmenorrhea: A Randomized Clinical Trial," *Oman Medical Journal* 32, no. 1 (2017): 47–53, https://doi.org/10.5001/omj.2017.09.

153 **menstrual periods disrupt:** Hassan Nagy, Karen Carlson, and Moien A.B. Khan, "Dysmenorrhea," StatPearls, last updated November 12, 2023, https://www.ncbi.nlm.nih.gov/books/NBK560834/.

153 **70 percent of menstruating people:** Irene O. Aninye, Melissa H. Laitner, and Society for Women's Health Research Uterine Fibroids Working Group, "Uterine Fibroids: Assessing Unmet Needs from Bench to Bedside," *Journal of Women's Health* 30, no. 8 (2021): 1060–67, https://doi.org/10.1089/jwh.2021.0280.

153 **Up to 12 percent:** "PCOS (Polycystic Ovary Syndrome) and Diabetes," Centers for Disease Control and Prevention, last updated December 30, 2022, https://www.cdc.gov/diabetes/basics/pcos.html.

154 **More than 11 percent:** "Endometriosis," Office on Women's Health, last updated February 22, 2021, https://www.womenshealth.gov/a-z-topics/endometriosis.

154 **tissue grows outside of the uterus:** Aalia Sachedina and Nicole Todd, "Dysmenorrhea, Endometriosis and Chronic Pelvic Pain in Adolescents," *Journal of Clinical Research in Pediatric Endocrinology* 12, suppl. 1 (2020): 7–17, https://doi.org/10.4274/jcrpe.galenos.2019.2019.S0217.

154 **About 10 percent of people:** Victoria Pelham, "Understanding Ovarian Cysts," *Cedars-Sinai Blog,* April 4, 2022, https://www.cedars-sinai.org/blog/treating-ovarian-cysts.html.

154 **eat more sugar and drink:** Nastaran Najafi et al., "Major Dietary Patterns in Relation to Menstrual Pain: A Nested Case Control Study," *BMC Women's Health* 18, no. 1 (2018):69, https://doi.org/10.1186/s12905-018-0558-4.

154 **up to 90 percent:** Robert L. Reid, "Premenstrual Dysphoric Disorder (Formerly Premenstrual Syndrome)," Endotext, last updated January 23, 2017, https://www.ncbi.nlm.nih.gov/books/NBK279045/.

155 **premenstrual dysphoric disorder (PMDD):** M. Steiner, "Premenstrual Syndrome and Premenstrual Dysphoric Disorder: Guidelines for Management," *Journal of Psychiatry and Neuroscience* 25, no. 5 (2000): 459–68, https://www.ncbi.nlm.nih.gov/pmc/articles/PMC1408015.

155 **exercise for natural:** Motahari-Tabari, Shirvani, and Alipour, "Comparison of the Effect of Stretching Exercises."

155 **rule out more serious illnesses:** "Premenstrual Dysphoric Disorder (PMDD)," Johns Hopkins Medicine, November 19, 2019, https://www.hopkinsmedicine.org/health/conditions-and-diseases/premenstrual-dysphoric-disorder-pmdd.

155 **Menstrual cycles tend to continue:** "Your Menstrual Cycle," Office on Women's Health, last updated February 22, 2021, https://www.womenshealth.gov/menstrual-cycle/your-menstrual-cycle.

155 **changed often to prevent:** "Pads vs. Tampons: What to Know," WebMD, last updated August 12, 2023, https://www.webmd.com/women/pads-vs-tampons-what-to-know.

156 **made of absorbent materials:** "Pads vs. Tampons," WebMD.

156 **made of sturdier fabrics:** Sara Coughlin, "So You Want to Board the Reusable Pad Bandwagon," *Self*, September 16, 2020, https://www.self.com/story/reusable-pads.

156 **designed to hold more blood:** Kim Schneider, "What Is Period Underwear and Does It Work?," *Health Essentials* (blog), Cleveland Clinic, February 7, 2022, https://health.clevelandclinic.org/does-period-underwear-work/.

156 **longer than twelve hours:** Schneider, "What Is Period Underwear?"

156 **mix of cotton and:** "The Facts on Tampons—and How to Use Them Safely," US Food and Drug Administration, September 30, 2020. https://www.fda.gov/consumers/consumer-updates/facts-tampons-and-how-use-them-safely.

157 **changed every four to eight hours:** "The Facts on Tampons," U.S. Food and Drug Administration.

157 **cup shape once inside:** Annamarya Scaccia, "Everything You Need to Know about Using Menstrual Cups," Healthline, last updated April 9, 2019, https://www.healthline.com/health/womens-health/menstrual-cup.

157 **reusable after washing:** Scaccia, "Everything You Need to Know."

157 **discs work like cups:** Adrienne Santos-Longhurst, "Are Menstrual Discs the Period Product We've Been Waiting For?," Healthline, February 10, 2020, https://www.healthline.com/health/menstrual-disc#insertion.

157 **extra capacity and barely there:** Santos-Longhurst, "Menstrual Discs?"

157 **toxic shock syndrome (TSS):** "Streptococcal Toxic Shock Syndrome: All You Need to Know," Centers for Disease Control and Prevention, last updated June 27, 2022, https://www.cdc.gov/groupastrep/diseases-public/streptococcal-toxic-shock-syndrome.html.

157 **The longer you wait:** Kristen Domonell, "Toxic Shock Syndrome Is Rare. Here's What Tampon Users Should Know," Right as Rain by UW Medicine, March 7, 2018, https://rightasrain.uwmedicine.org/well/health/toxic-shock-syndrome-rare-heres-what-tampon-users-should-know.

157 **Alternating between internal and external:** "Staph Infections," Mayo Clinic, accessed January 9, 2024, https://www.mayoclinic.org/diseases-conditions/staph-infections/symptoms-causes/syc-20356221?p=1.

157 **having flu-like symptoms:** "Toxic Shock Syndrome," Mayo Clinic, last updated March 23, 2022, https://www.mayoclinic.org/diseases-conditions/toxic-shock-syndrome/symptoms-causes/syc-20355384.

158 **supposed to be moist:** "Vaginal Discharge," Mayo Clinic, April 25, 2023, https://www.mayoclinic.org/symptoms/vaginal-discharge/basics/definition/sym-20050825.

158 **indicate various phases:** "Cervical Mucus," Cleveland Clinic, last updated October 24, 2021, https://my.clevelandclinic.org/health/body/21957-cervical-mucus.

158 **something being awry:** "Vaginal Discharge," Cleveland Clinic, last updated July 22, 2022, https://my.clevelandclinic.org/health/symptoms/4719-vaginal-discharge.

158 **vaginal discharge matches:** "Vaginal Discharge," Mayo Clinic.

158 **teaspoon a day:** D. A. Eschenbach et al., "Influence of the Normal Menstrual Cycle on Vaginal Tissue, Discharge, and Microflora," *Clinical Infectious Diseases* 30, no. 6 (2000): 901–907, doi: 10.1086/313818.

159 **born with vaginas get BV:** "Bacterial Vaginosis," Cleveland Clinic, last updated February 6, 2023, https://my.clevelandclinic.org/health/diseases/3963-bacterial-vaginosis.

160 **what the discharge does:** "Cervical Mucus," Cleveland Clinic.

160 **calendars often had thirteen months:** "History of the 13-Month Calendar," in *Journal of Calendar Reform XVI*, no. 4 (1944): 165–66. https://myweb.ecu.edu/mccartyr/13-month.htm.

161 **cleaning inside the vaginal canal:** "Cervical Mucus," Cleveland Clinic.

161 **does not prevent STIs:** "Safer Sex Guidelines for Teens," Stanford Medicine Children's Health, accessed January 9, 2024, https://www.stanfordchildrens.org/en/topic/default?id=safer-sex-guidelines-for-adolescents-90-P01645.

161 **vaginas who douche:** Kim Schneider, "Why You Should Never Douche," *Health Essentials* (blog), Cleveland Clinic, July 26, 2022, https://health.clevelandclinic.org/douche/.

161 **as well as abnormal discharge:** Didem Sunay, Erdal Kaya, and Yusuf Ergün, "Vaginal Douching Behavior of Women and Relationship among Vaginal Douching and Vaginal Discharge and Demographic Factors," *Journal of Turkish Society of Obstetrics and Gynecology* 8, no. 4 (2011): 264–67, https://doi.org/10.5505/tjod.2011.57805.

Sex, Gender & Sexual Health

164 **one of the categories:** NIH Style Guide, "Sex, Gender, and Sexuality," National Institutes of Health (NIH), last updated November 14, 2023, https://www.nih.gov/nih-style-guide/sex-gender-sexuality.

164 **Some places allow:** "Non-Binary Birth Certificates and State IDs: Full Guide," US Birth Certificates, last updated May 30, 2023, https://www.usbirthcertificates

.com/articles/gender-neutral-birth
-certificates-states.

164 **Hormones are chemicals:** "Hormones,"
MedlinePlus, October 7, 2016, https://
medlineplus.gov/hormones.html.

164 **called sex hormones:** Sarah Sistek,
"Changes Ahead: Talking with Children about
Puberty," *Speaking of Health* (blog), Mayo
Clinic Health System, October 25, 2022,
https://www.mayoclinichealthsystem.org
/hometown-health/speaking-of-health
/talking-with-children-about-puberty.

165 **puberty starts (often:** "About Puberty
and Precocious Puberty," Eunice Kennedy
Shriver National Institute of Child Health
and Human Development, last updated
June 21, 2021, https://www.nichd.nih.gov
/health/topics/puberty/conditioninfo.

165 **"male" sex traits:** Logan Breehl and Omar
Caban, "Physiology, Puberty," StatPearls,
last updated March 27, 2023, https://www
.ncbi.nlm.nih.gov/books/NBK534827.

165 **"female" sex traits:** Breehl and Caban,
"Physiology, Puberty."

165 **An intersex variation is any type:**
"What's Intersex?" Planned Parenthood,
accessed January 9, 2024, https://www
.plannedparenthood.org/learn/gender
-identity/sex-gender-identity/whats
-intersex.

165 **in the womb, the same tissue:** "Ambiguous
Genitalia," MedlinePlus, last updated April
25, 2023, https://medlineplus.gov/ency
/article/003269.htm.

166 **around 1.7 percent:** Laetitia Zeeman and
Kay Aranda, "A Systematic Review of
the Health and Healthcare Inequalities
for People with Intersex Variance,"
*International Journal of Environmental
Research and Public Health* 17, no. 18
(2020): 6533, https://doi.org/10.3390
/ijerph17186533.

166 **born with green eyes:** Steph Coelho, "What
Is the Rarest Eye Color?," Verywell Health,
last updated March 12, 2023, https://www
.verywellhealth.com/what-is-the-rarest
-eye-color-5087302.

166 **people worldwide have vitiligo:** Prathmesh
Nimkar and Anil Wanjari, "Vitiligo and the
Role of Newer Therapeutic Modalities,"
Cureus 14, no. 11 (2022): e31022, https://
doi.org/10.7759/cureus.31022.

166 **inflammatory bowel disease:** Gian
Paolo Caviglia et al., "Epidemiology
of Inflammatory Bowel Diseases: A
Population Study in a Healthcare District
of North-West Italy," *Journal of Clinical
Medicine* 12, no. 12 (2023): 641, https://doi
.org/10.3390/jcm12020641.

166 **have red hair:** Andrew Cunningham et al.,
"Red for Danger: The Effects of Red Hair in
Surgical Practice," *BMJ* 341 (2010): c6931,
https://doi.org/10.1136/bmj.c6931.

166 **have juvenile diabetes:** "Statistics About
Diabetes," American Diabetes Association,
accessed January 9, 2024, https://
diabetes.org/about-diabetes/statistics
/about-diabetes.

167 **Gender identity is how you feel:** NIH Style
Guide, "Sex, Gender, and Sexuality."

168 **The term** *nonbinary:* "Understanding
Nonbinary People: How to Be Respectful
and Supportive," National Center for
Transgender Equality, January 12, 2023,
https://transequality.org/issues/resources
/understanding-nonbinary-people-how-to
-be-respectful-and-supportive.

169 **gender inclusive alternatives:** Jennifer E.
Arnold, Heather C. Mayo, and Lisa Dong,
"My Pronouns Are *They/Them*: Talking
about Pronouns Changes How Pronouns
Are Understood," *Psychonomic Bulletin
and Review* 28, no. 5 (2021): 1688–97,
https://doi.org/10.3758/s13423-021
-01905-0.

169 experiencing gender dysphoria: Garmina Garg, Ghada Elshimy, and Raman Marwaha, "Gender Dysphoria," StatPearls, last updated July 11, 2023, https://www.ncbi.nlm.nih.gov/books/NBK532313/.

170 called gender expression: NIH Style Guide, "Sex, Gender, and Sexuality."

171 access to gender-affirming care: Elliott David Jr., "States That Have Restricted Gender-Affirming Care for Trans Youth in 2023," *US News and World Report*, last updated January 5, 2024, https://www.usnews.com/news/best-states/articles/2023-03-30/what-is-gender-affirming-care-and-which-states-have-restricted-it-in-2023.

171 gametes of people: Martha Lally and Suzanne Valentine-French, "Sexual Development," in Chapter 6 of *Lifespan Development: A Psychological Perspective,* 2nd ed. (2019): 216, https://courses.lumenlearning.com/suny-lifespandevelopment/chapter/sexual-development.

171 produce and store sperm: "Gamete," Scitable by Nature Education, accessed January 9, 2024, https://www.nature.com/scitable/definition/gamete-gametes-311.

171 embryo, which can eventually grow: "Conception," Cleveland Clinic, last updated September 6, 2022, https://my.clevelandclinic.org/health/articles/11585-conception.

171 can reproduce year-round: Bogusław Pawłowski and Andrzej Żelaźniewicz, "The Evolution of Perennially Enlarged Breasts in Women: A Critical Review and a Novel Hypothesis," *Biological Reviews* 96, no. 6 (2021): 2794–809, https://doi.org/10.1111/brv.12778.

172 develops during puberty: Anna Kågesten and Miranda van Reeuwijk, "Healthy Sexuality Development in Adolescence: Proposing a Competency-Based Framework to Inform Programmes and Research," *Sexual and Reproductive Health Matters* 29, no. 1 (2021): 19961116, https://www.ncbi.nlm.nih.gov/pmc/articles/PMC8725766/.

174 sexually active by the time they're twenty: Marina Epstein et al., "Adolescent Age of Sexual Initiation and Subsequent Adult Health Outcomes," *American Journal of Public Health* 108, no. 6 (2018): 822–28, https://doi.org/10.2105/ajph.2018.304372.

174 (yes, ten) important things to know: "Safer Sex," Stanford Medicine Children's Health.

174 asking for permission: "What Consent Looks Like," RAINN, accessed January 9, 2024, https://www.rainn.org/articles/what-is-consent.

174 know the truth: "Sexual Consent," Planned Parenthood, accessed January 9, 2024, https://www.plannedparenthood.org/learn/relationships/sexual-consent.

176 through skin-to-skin contact: "STDs," Planned Parenthood, https://www.plannedparenthood.org/learn/stds-hiv-safer-sex/hpv.

177 PrEP (pre-exposure prophylaxis): "Pre-Exposure Prophylaxis (PrEP)," HIV Risk and Prevention, Centers for Disease Control and Prevention, last updated July 5, 2022, https://www.cdc.gov/hiv/risk/prep/index.html.

178 Outercourse, such as: "Abstinence and Outercourse," Planned Parenthood, accessed January 9, 2024, https://www.plannedparenthood.org/learn/birth-control/abstinence-and-outercourse.

178 toys can also transmit STIs: Jeanne M. Marrazzo, Patricia Coffey, and Allison Bingham, "Sexual Practices, Risk Perception and Knowledge of Sexually Transmitted Disease Risk among Lesbian and Bisexual Women," *Perspectives on*

Sexual and Reproductive Health 37, no. 1 (2005): 6–12, https://doi.org/10.1363/psrh.37.006.05.

179 **Internal condoms are:** "Obstetrical and Gynecological Devices; Reclassification of Single-Use Female Condom, to Be Renamed Single-Use Internal Condom," *Federal Register,* September 27, 2018, https://www.federalregister.gov/documents/2018/09/27/2018-21044/obstetrical-and-gynecological-devices-reclassification-of-single-use-female-condom-to-be-renamed.

179 **put on an external condom:** "How to Put a Condom On," Planned Parenthood, accessed January 9, 2024, https://www.plannedparenthood.org/learn/birth-control/condom/how-to-put-a-condom-on.

180 **"double bagging" condoms:** Heba Mahdy, Ari D. Shaeffer, Daniel M. McNabb, "Condoms," StatPearls, last updated April 17, 2023, https://www.ncbi.nlm.nih.gov/books/NBK470385/.

181 **While a dental dam:** Daniel Gutierrez et al., "Dental Dams in Dermatology: An Underutilized Barrier Method of Protection," *International Journal of Women's Dermatology* 8, no. 1 (2022): e008, https://doi.org/10.1097/jw9.0000000000000008/.

181 **household plastic wrap:** "STD Awareness: Can I Use Plastic Wrap as a Dental Dam During Oral Sex?," Planned Parenthood Action Fund, January 4, 2016, https://www.plannedparenthoodaction.org/planned-parenthood-advocates-arizona/blog/std-awareness-can-i-use-plastic-wrap-as-a-dental-dam-during-oral-sex.

181 **Permanent birth control:** "Sterilization as a Family Planning Method," KFF, December 14, 2018, https://www.kff.org/womens-health-policy/fact-sheet/sterilization-as-a-family-planning-method/.

181 **paired with condom usage:** Liz Seegert, "When to Use Backup Birth Control," WebMD, June 11, 2022, https://www.webmd.com/sex/birth-control/backup-birth-control.

182 **failure rate can be up to 13 percent:** "How Effective Are Condoms?," Planned Parenthood, accessed January 9, 2024, https://www.plannedparenthood.org/learn/birth-control/condom/how-effective-are-condoms.

182 **When used alone, diaphragms fail:** "Contraception," Centers for Disease Control and Prevention, last updated May 1, 2023, https://www.cdc.gov/reproductivehealth/contraception/index.htm.

183 **The implant fails:** "Contraception," Centers for Disease Control and Prevention.

183 **The patch fails:** ""Contraception," Centers for Disease Control and Prevention.

183 **The ring fails:** "Contraception," Centers for Disease Control and Prevention.

183 **The shot fails:** "Contraception," Centers for Disease Control and Prevention.

183 **The IUD fails:** "Contraception," Centers for Disease Control and Prevention.

184 **21 out of every 100:** "Contraception," Centers for Disease Control and Prevention.

184 **forms of emergency contraception:** "Emergency Contraception," World Health Organization, November 9, 2021, https://www.who.int/news-room/fact-sheets/detail/emergency-contraception.

184 **having an IUD:** "How Do IUDs Work as Emergency Contraception?," Planned Parenthood, accessed January 9, 2024, https://www.plannedparenthood.org

/learn/morning-after-pill-emergency
-contraception/how-do-iuds-work
-emergency-contraception.

184 **morning-after pill is taken:** "Morning-After Pill," Mayo Clinic, June 3, 2022, https://www.mayoclinic.org/tests-procedures/morning-after-pill/about/pac-20394730.

184 **within three days of intercourse:** "Morning-After Pill," Mayo Clinic.

184 **weigh over 165 pounds:** Krishna K. Upadhya et al., "Emergency Contraception," *Pediatrics* 144, no. 6 (2019): e20193149, https://doi.org/10.1542/peds.2019-3149.

185 **1 in every 5 people has:** "Sexually Transmitted Infections Prevalence, Incidence, and Cost Estimates in the United States," Centers for Disease Control and Prevention, last updated January 25, 2021, https://www.cdc.gov/std/statistics/prevalence-2020-at-a-glance.htm.

185 **half of all new STIs:** "Sexually Transmitted Infections Workgroup," Healthy People 2030, accessed January 9, 2024, https://health.gov/healthypeople/about/work groups/sexually-transmitted-infections-workgroup.

185 **even kissing can spread:** "Safer Sex Guidelines," Johns Hopkins Medicine, accessed January 9, 2024, https://www.hopkinsmedicine.org/health/wellness-and-prevention/safer-sex-guidelines#:~:text=For%20example%2C%20kissing%20is%20thought,thought%20to%20protect%20against%20STIs.

185 **recognize any of the symptoms:** "Sexually Transmitted Disease (STD) Symptoms," Mayo Clinic, May 5, 2022, https://www.mayoclinic.org/diseases-conditions/sexually-transmitted-diseases-stds/in-depth/std-symptoms/art-20047081.

185 **report being sexually assaulted:** "Steps You Can Take after Sexual Assault," RAINN, accessed January 9, 2024, https://www

.rainn.org/articles/steps-you-can-take-after-sexual-assault.

186 **someone the person knows:** Ateret Gewirtz-Meydan and David Finkelhor, "Sexual Abuse and Assault in a Large National Sample of Children and Adolescents," *Child Maltreatment* 25, no. 2 (2020): 203–14, https://doi.org/10.1177/1077559519873975.

186 **the following steps after sexual assault:** "Emergency Medical Assistance and Preserving Evidence," MIT Institute Discrimination and Harassment Response Office, accessed January 9, 2024, https://idhr.mit.edu/reporting-options/emergency-medical.

186 **mental health support:** "Self-Care," Victim Connect Resource Center," May 6, 2021, https://victimconnect.org/learn/self-care/.

186 **victims may suffer:** Dean G. Kilpatrick, "Mental Health Impact of Rape," accessed January 9, 2024, https://mainweb-v.musc.edu/vawprevention/research/mental impact.shtml.

187 **sexual assault helpline:** RAINN, accessed January 9, 2024, https://www.rainn.org/.

Seeking Help & Self–Care

192 **see your PCP once a year:** "Choosing a Primary Care Provider," MedlinePlus, last updated July 8, 2023, https://medlineplus.gov/ency/article/001939.htm.

192 **Many types of medical professionals can serve:** "Primary Care Specialties," University of Mississippi Medical Center, accessed January 9, 2024, https://www.umc.edu/Healthcare/Primary%20Care/Primary-Care-Specialties.html.

194 **PCP can often refer:** Malhar P. Patel et al., "Closing the Referral Loop: An Analysis of Primary Care Referrals to Specialists in a Large Health System," *Journal of General*

Internal Medicine 33, no. 5 (2018): 715–21, https://doi.org/10.1007/s11606-018 -4392-z.

196 support that you trust: Rebecca Joy Stanborough, "How to Find a Therapist: 8 Tips for the Right Fit," Healthline, last updated November 14, 2023, https://www .healthline.com/health/how-to-find-a -therapist#insurance-directory.

197 a trained mental health professional: Linda Godleski, Adam Darkins, and John W. Peters, "Outcomes of 98,609 U.S. Department of Veterans Affairs Patients Enrolled in Telemental Health Services, 2006–2010," *Psychiatric Services* 63, no. 4 (2012): 383–85, https://doi.org/10.1176 /appi.ps.201100206.

198 Online talk therapy: "What You Need to Know Before Choosing Online Therapy," American Psychological Association, October 7, 2015, https://www.apa.org /topics/telehealth/online-therapy.

198 mental health medications: "Mental Health Medications," National Institute of Mental Health (NIMH), last updated December 2023, https://www.nimh.nih.gov/health /topics/mental-health-medications.

199 serious mental illness: "About Mental Health," Centers for Disease Control and Prevention, last updated April 25, 2023, https://www.cdc.gov/mentalhealth/learn /index.htm.

200 Depression. Unshakable feelings: Suma P. Chand and Hasan Arif, "Depression," StatPearls, last updated July 17, 2023, https://www.ncbi.nlm.nih.gov/books /NBK430847.

200 Unshakable feelings of fear: Suma P. Chand and Raman Marwaha, "Anxiety," StatPearls, last updated April 24, 2023, https://www.ncbi.nlm.nih.gov/books /NBK470361.

200 types of anxiety disorders: "Anxiety Disorders," Mayo Clinic, last updated May 4, 2018, https://www.mayoclinic.org /diseases-conditions/anxiety/symptoms -causes/syc-20350961.

201 cycle of reoccurring thoughts: "Obsessive-Compulsive Disorder," National Institute of Mental Health (NIMH), last updated September 2022, https://www.nimh.nih .gov/health/topics/obsessive-compulsive -disorder-ocd.

201 6 percent of the population: "Post-Traumatic Stress Disorder," National Institute of Mental Health (NIMH), last updated May 2023, https://www.nimh.nih .gov/health/topics/post-traumatic-stress -disorder-ptsd.

201 Body dysmorphic disorder: Holly R. Nicewicz and Jacqueline F. Boutrouille, "Body Dysmorphic Disorder," StatPearls, last updated September 28, 2022, https:// www.ncbi.nlm.nih.gov/books/NBK555901.

202 Eating disorders. When: "Eating Disorders: About More Than Food," National Institute of Mental Health (NIMH), last updated 2021, https://www.nimh.nih.gov/health /publications/eating-disorders.

202 avoidant restrictive food intake disorder (ARFID): Agata Kozak et al., "Avoidant/ Restrictive Food Disorder (ARFID), Food Neophobia, Other Eating-Related Behaviours and Feeding Practices among Children with Autism Spectrum Disorder and in Non-Clinical Sample: A Preliminary Study," *International Journal of Environmental Research and Public Health* 20, no. 10 (2023): 5822, https://doi .org/10.3390/ijerph20105822.

202 lack the ability to control: "Substance Use and Co-Occurring Mental Disorders," National Institute of Mental Health (NIMH), last updated March 2023, https://www .nimh.nih.gov/health/topics/substance -use-and-mental-health.

202 Americans over the age of twelve: "SAMHSA Announces National Survey on Drug Use and Health (NSDUH) Results Detailing Mental Illness and Substance Use Levels in 2021," Substance Abuse and Mental Health Services Administration (SAMHSA), January 4, 2023, https://www.hhs.gov/about/news/2023/01/04/samhsa-announces-national-survey-drug-use-health-results-detailing-mental-illness-substance-use-levels-2021.

202 Attention-deficit/hyperactivity disorder: "Attention-Deficit/Hyperactivity Disorder," National Institute of Mental Health (NIMH), last updated September 2023, https://www.nimh.nih.gov/health/topics/attention-deficit-hyperactivity-disorder-adhd.

202 13 percent of teenagers: "Data and Statistics about ADHD," Centers for Disease Control and Prevention, last updated October 16, 2023, https://www.cdc.gov/ncbddd/adhd/data.html.

203 1 in 5 people worldwide: Donna Gillies et al., "Prevalence and Characteristics of Self-Harm in Adolescents: Meta-Analyses of Community-Based Studies 1990–2015," *Journal of the American Academy of Child and Adolescent Psychiatry* 57, no. 10 (2018): 733–41, https://doi.org/10.1016/j.jaac.2018.06.018.

203 people who self-harm: Martin A. Monto, Nick McRee, and Frank S. Deryck, "Nonsuicidal Self-Injury among a Representative Sample of US Adolescents, 2015," *American Journal of Public Health* 108, no. 8 (2018): 1042–48, https://doi.org/10.2105/ajph.2018.304470.

203 considering ending their own life: Farzana Akkas, "Youth Suicide Risk Increased over Past Decade," Pew Charitable Trusts, March 3, 2023, https://www.pewtrusts.org/en/research-and-analysis/articles/2023/03/03/youth-suicide-risk-increased-over-past-decade.

203 More than 20 percent of high school students: "988 Suicide and Crisis Lifeline Adds Spanish Text and Chat Service Ahead of One-Year Anniversary," Substance Abuse and Mental Health Services Administration (SAMHSA), July 13, 2023, https://www.samhsa.gov/newsroom/press-announcements/20230713/988-suicide-crisis-lifeline-adds-spanish-text-chat-service-ahead-one-year-anniversary.

203 speaking with a trained counselor: Home page, 988 Suicide and Crisis Lifeline, accessed January 9, 2024, https://988lifeline.org.

205 Self-care is the lifelong process: "Caring for Your Mental Health," National Institute of Mental Health (NIMH), last updated December 2022, https://www.nimh.nih.gov/health/topics/caring-for-your-mental-health.

205 better mental health and body image: "Reducing Social Media Use Significantly Improves Body Image in Teens, Young Adults: Participants Saw Results in Weeks, Study Says," ScienceDaily, February 23, 2023, https://www.sciencedaily.com/releases/2023/02/230223132843.htm.

206 eight and ten hours each night: Jennifer Bowers and Anne Moyer, "Adolescent Sleep and Technology-Use Rules: Results from the California Health Interview Survey," *Sleep Health* 6, no. 1 (2020): 19–22, https://doi.org/10.1016/j.sleh.2019.08.011.

206 sleep is crucial: Alexander J. Scott et al., "Improving Sleep Quality Leads to Better Mental Health: A Meta-Analysis of Randomised Controlled Trials," *Sleep Medicine Reviews* 60 (2021): 101556, https://doi.org/10.1016/j.smrv.2021.101556.

206 Thirty minutes a day: "Caring for Your Mental Health," NIMH.

206 **an hour of exercise:** "Physical Activity Guidelines for School-Aged Children and Adolescents," Centers for Disease Control and Prevention, last updated July 26, 2022, https://www.cdc.gov/healthyschools /physicalactivity/guidelines.htm.

206 **strengthens your body and releases endorphins:** Yun Jun Yang, "An Overview of Current Physical Activity Recommendations in Primary Care," *Korean Journal of Family Medicine* 40, no. 3 (2019): 135–42, https://doi.org/ 10.4082/kjfm.19.0038.

206 **interesting pursuits can give:** "Self-Care: 5 Ways to Take Good Care of Yourself," Geisinger, December 21, 2021, https:// www.geisinger.org/health-and-wellness /wellness-articles/2021/01/11/16/10/5 -self-care-tips.

206 **You can't prevent every single accident:** Canadian Paediatric Society, "Injury Prevention Tips for Healthy Active Living at Home, School and in the Community," *Paediatrics and Child Health* 7, no. 5 (2002): 304–306, https://www.ncbi.nlm .nih.gov/pmc/articles/PMC2795617/.

207 **damage from abusing these substances:** "Drug Misuse and Addiction," National Institute on Drug Abuse, July 13, 2020, https://nida.nih.gov/publications/drugs -brains-behavior-science-addiction/drug -misuse-addiction.

207 **yoga, or meditating:** Emily Cronkleton, "Here's How to Use Yoga for Stress Reduction," Healthline, May 4, 2021, https://www.healthline.com/health /fitness/yoga-for-stress.

207 **eating lots of high-fiber foods:** "Does What You Eat Affect Your Mood?," *Health Essentials* (blog), Cleveland Clinic, last updated January 12, 2021, https://health .clevelandclinic.org/bad-mood-look-to -your-food/.

208 **at least eight hours of sleep:** Anne G. Wheaton et al., "Short Sleep Duration among Middle School and High School Students—United States, 2015," *Morbidity and Mortality Weekly Report* 67, no. 3 (2018): 85–90, https://doi.org/10.15585 /mmwr.mm6703a.

208 **better sleep can improve:** Alexander J. Scott et al., "Improving Sleep Quality Leads to Better Mental Health: A Meta-Analysis of Randomised Controlled Trials," *Sleep Medicine Reviews* 60 (2021): 101556. https://doi.org/10.1016/j.smrv.2021.101556.

209 **messes with your sleep:** Nazish Rafique et al., "Effects of Mobile Use on Subjective Sleep Quality," *Nature and Science of Sleep* 12 (2020): 357–64, https://doi.org/10.2147 /nss.s253375.

210 **8 percent of teens and young adults:** Graciela E. Silva et al., "Restless Legs Syndrome, Sleep, and Quality of Life among Adolescents and Young Adults," *Journal of Clinical Sleep Medicine* 10, no. 7 (2014): 779–86, https://doi.org/10.5664 /jcsm.3872.

credits

All photographs featured in *The Real Body Manual* were taken by Brynne Zaniboni (www.brynnezaniboni.com) except the following:

index

Note: Italicized page numbers indicate material in tables or illustrations.

hormones *(continued)*
    and hair loss, 60
    hormone therapy, 171
    imbalances in, 56–57
    and menstrual cycles, 86
    and puberty, 164
"hot tub" folliculitis, 25
human immunodeficiency virus
    (HIV), 177
human papillomavirus (HPV)
    and bumps/lumps around
        anus, 98
    testing for, 27
    vaccine for, 176–77
    and warts, 26, 127
hygiene practices, 206. *See
    also* bathing/showering
hyperhidrosis, 4, 6, 8
hyperpigmentation, 38–39,
    154
hypodermis/subcutaneous
    tissues, 3
hypopigmentation, 36–37
hypospadias, 130

i
illness, 6
implanted birth control, 182–83
impotence (erectile
    dysfunction), 142–43
incontinence, 108
infections and body odors, 123
inflammatory bowel disease
    (IBD), 114
ingrown hairs, 24, 65–66
ingrown nails, 45–46
injury prevention, 206
intersex people
    about, 165
    and breast tissue, 79, 81
    developmental variations of,
        120, 165–66
    and douching, 161
    and gender identity, 168
    prevalence of, 166
    and sex assignments at
        birth, 164

and terms relating to
    genitalia, xi
intertrigo, 42
intestines, 101. *See also* bowels
intrauterine devices (IUDs),
    183, 184
irritable bowel syndrome (IBS),
    114
IUDs (birth control), 183, 184

j
jewelry, 22
jock itch, 42–43, 121, 123

k
keloids, 34
kidney stones, 110
kissing, 18, 185

l
labia, *145*
    anatomy of, 144
    and Bartholin's cysts, 122,
        144, 147
    as erogenous zone, 146
    and smegma, 126
    surgeries to reduce, 124, 125
    washing, 13, 14
laxatives, 101
legs, 13, 31–32
lesbians, 172–73
lice, 48, 49, 66
lips
    chapped, 17
    hair growing on, 56–57
    sores on, 17–18, 128
    and sun protection, 29
lubricants and painful
    urination, 109

m
Māhū (Hawaii), 167
makeup, 23
mammals (term), 70
mammary glands, 70
manicures with UV lights, 31
massage, 178

masturbation
    achieving orgasm with, 146
    and cramping, 153
    and penile fractures, 141
    self-masturbating together,
        178
medical professionals, 192–95
medical sterilization, 181
medications from other people,
    207
melanocytes, 38
melanoma, 45
menopause, 155
menorrhagia, 149–50
menstrual cycles, 148–57
    about, 148
    blood expelled in, 149
    and blood in stool, 95
    and constipation, 97
    and cramping, 152–54
    and discharge from vagina,
        158, 160
    discomfort associated with,
        148
    duration of, 160
    fluctuations in, 149
    frequency of, 152
    heavy periods, 149–50
    and hormonal birth control,
        151
    and intersex people, 166
    and lumpy breasts, 86
    and menopause, 155
    missing periods, 150–51
    and ovaries' egg production,
        171
    and PMS/PMDD, 154–55
    and preventing unplanned
        pregnancies, 177
    products for managing,
        155–57
    tracking, 152
mental health issues
    anxiety, 8, 199, 200, 203
    body dysmorphic disorder, 201
    depression, 14, 199, 200,
        203